Atlas of Breast Lesions on Chest Computed Tomography

Afsaneh Alikhassi

Atlas of Breast Lesions on Chest Computed Tomography

Springer

Afsaneh Alikhassi
Medical Imaging, Sunnybrook
Health Science Centre
University of Toronto
Toronto, ON, Canada

ISBN 978-3-032-22790-4 ISBN 978-3-032-22791-1 (eBook)
https://doi.org/10.1007/978-3-032-22791-1

This Springer imprint is published by the registered company Springer Nature Switzerland AG
The registered company address is: Gewerbestrasse 11, 6330 Cham, Switzerland

To my husband, Keivan, and my daughter, Rosha

Preface

Chest CT is typically used for diagnosing lung, mediastinum, pleura, and chest wall conditions, but it can also detect breast abnormalities, including cancer. With the increased use of chest CT, incidental breast lesions are increasingly being detected. In some cases, chest CT may be the first imaging modality to demonstrate breast cancer.

Chest CT is not the preferred method for characterizing breast lesions. However, radiologists frequently encounter breast lesions in chest CT scans, particularly with high-quality images from newer CT scan machines. Unlike mammography, ultrasound, and MRI, there is no standardized set of descriptors for CT scans in the Breast Imaging Reporting and Data System.

While chest CT scans offer advantages such as comfort and no need for compression, there are concerns about overuse and radiation risks associated with CT scans in general.

As CT technology evolves, there is an opportunity to refine protocols for using chest CT scans in breast cancer screening. This includes optimizing radiation doses and improving radiologist training to enhance detection rates for incidental cancers.

This book aims to illustrate various breast lesions observed in chest CT scans, showcasing both typical and atypical examples in each section. We have discussed some of the most critical types of breast lesions across five chapters. The images included have been carefully selected, and we hope this atlas serves as a valuable resource for radiology residents, fellows, general radiologists, radiologists specializing in thoracic imaging, and clinicians. Ultimately, this resource may contribute to the earlier detection of breast cancer and improve patients' breast health.

Toronto, ON, Canada — Afsaneh Alikhassi

Acknowledgments

I would like to express my heartfelt gratitude to those who have supported me on this journey. To my husband, whose steadfast support, patience, and encouragement have been invaluable throughout the process of writing this book. Your strength and understanding have been a constant source of motivation, and without you, this accomplishment would not have been possible. To my daughter, whose presence brings light, joy, and inspiration to my life. You remind me every day of the true purpose behind my efforts. I am also grateful to my colleagues and mentors, whose insights and expertise have enriched this work. Thank you all for believing in me and for helping make this atlas a reality.

Contents

Abbreviations

CHF	Congestive heart failure
CT	Computed tomography
DIEP flap	Deep Inferior Epigastric Perforator flap
3D	Three-dimensional
ER	Estrogen
GATA3	GATA binding protein 3
HU	Hansfield number
Her2	Human Epidermal Growth Factor Receptor 2
IBC	Inflammatory breast cancer
MIP	Maximum Intensity Projection
PASH	Pseudoangiomatous stromal hyperplasia
PR	Progesterone
RECIST	Response Evaluation Criteria in Solid Tumors
SCC	Squamous cell carcinoma
TRAM flap	Transverse rectus abdominis muscle flap
TTF1 receptor	Thyroid Transcription Factor-1
US	ultrasound

Chapter 1
Chest CT Findings of Malignant Breast Lesions

Radiologists need to be vigilant for the possibility of breast cancer when reviewing chest CT scans to avoid missing any cancer. The most common finding in the breast during chest CT scans is a mass [1]. Certain CT features, such as irregular shapes, non-circumscribed margins, and significant contrast enhancement, are indicators that may predict malignancy in incidental breast cancer cases [2–4]. Elise Desperito et al. reported that chest CT exceeded their expectations in terms of sensitivity, specificity, and accuracy for breast cancer diagnosis [1]. They found that chest CT scans, with or without contrast, demonstrated similar outcomes for specificity and accuracy in diagnosing breast cancer; however, sensitivity was slightly lower without IV contrast. Additionally, they noted that the false-negative rates for chest CT scans were comparable to those of mammography, while mammography had a higher number of false-positive exams. This discrepancy is likely due to the three-dimensional nature of CT scans, which minimizes the summation tissue effect seen in mammography. However, Bach et al. reported that distinguishing between benign and malignant breast lesions on chest CT is often unreliable. Circumscribed or weakly enhancing masses on chest CT can also be malignant [5]. This may be attributed to the larger field of view provided by chest CT, which results in less detailed imaging compared to breast MRI [2, 5].

Currently, there is no standardized CT lexicon specifically designed for breast imaging; however, the Breast Imaging Reporting and Data System (BI-RADS) terminology, used for mammography and MRI, can be adapted for this purpose. It is essential to use clear and descriptive terminology when categorizing abnormal findings in the breast during chest CT scan evaluations. To accurately describe CT-detected incidental findings in the breast, I recommend including the following details: whether the finding is a mass or non-mass; if it is markedly enhanced, or weakly/nonenhanced; the shape of the mass; whether it is irregular or oval/round; its size; whether it is unifocal or multifocal; and the presence of associated findings such as microcalcifications, nipple retraction, skin thickening, or enlarged axillary or internal mammary lymph nodes that may suggest metastatic involvement.

A. Alikhassi, *Atlas of Breast Lesions on Chest Computed Tomography*,
https://doi.org/10.1007/978-3-032-22791-1_1

Additionally, in our case descriptions, we compared the density of the mass with the surrounding normal fibroglandular tissue rather than with fat. Chest CT scans might be unable to recognize microcalcifications in breast mass; this issue could be tackled with a dedicated breast CT scan with a smaller field of view.

Finally, identifying specific CT features associated with incidental breast cancers may aid in developing artificial intelligence systems designed to accurately detect breast cancer on chest CT scans. Ultimately, this could lead to improved breast cancer diagnoses and better outcomes for patients.

Figures 1.1, 1.2, 1.3, 1.4, 1.5, 1.6, 1.7, 1.8, 1.9, 1.10, 1.11, 1.12, 1.13, 1.14, 1.15, 1.16, 1.17, 1.18, 1.19, and 1.20 describe the detection of malignant breast lesions on chest CT scans.

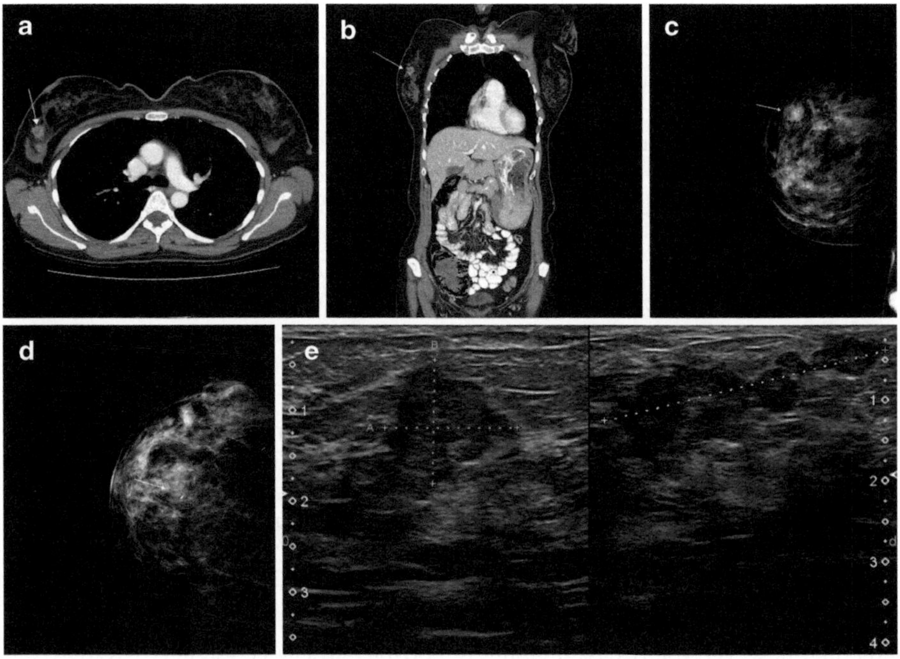

Fig. 1.1 Breast cancer in different modalities. Chest CT scan with IV contrast shows axial (**a**) and coronal reconstruction (**b**) views. Mammography was performed with MLO view (**c**) and CC view (**d**). Grayscale ultrasound (**e**), T1 sequence fat-suppressed axial MRI with contrast (**f**), and T1 sequence fat-suppressed late-phase sagittal MRI with contrast (**g**). The chest CT reveals an irregular-shape mass with spiculated borders and thick irregular rim enhancement, and central low density located in the right upper outer breast (arrow). Mammography demonstrates a partially obscured mass that is better seen in the MLO view than in the CC view, associated with a marker clip. Ultrasound confirmed the presence of an irregular mass with spiculated borders. MRI illustrates similar findings to chest CT scan. Additionally, a smaller, similar spiculated mass connected to the main mass and located posterosuperior to it was detected on the MRI. An ultrasound-guided biopsy confirmed the presence of invasive ductal carcinoma

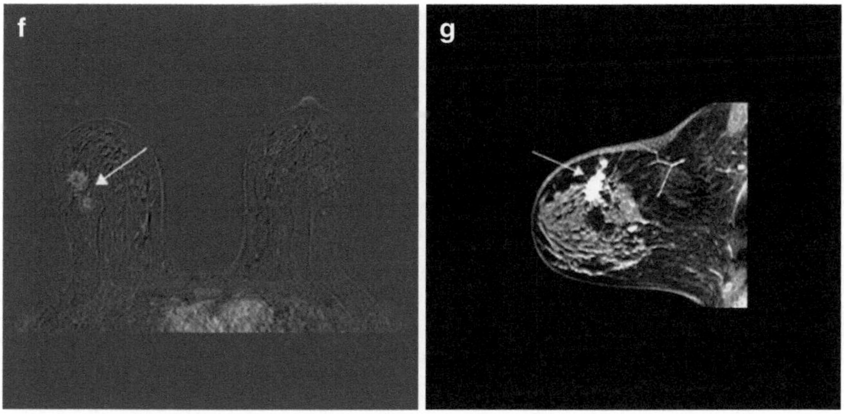

Fig. 1.1 (continued)

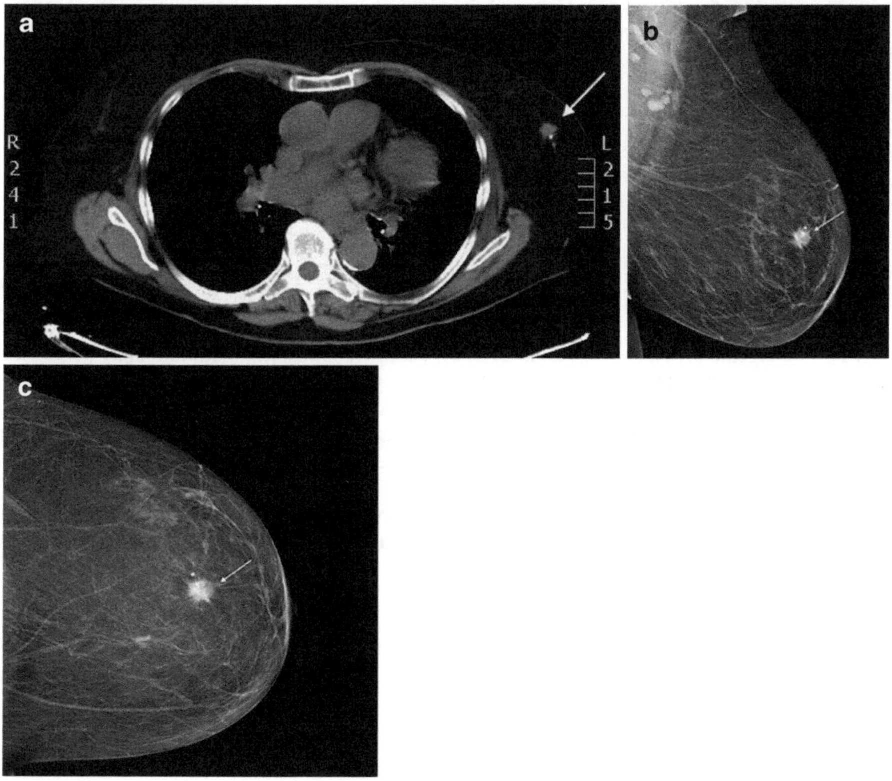

Fig. 1.2 Typical breast cancer in chest CT without IV contrast. Axial CT chest without IV contrast (**a**), mammography MLO view (**b**), and CC view (**c**). Chest CT scan demonstrates an irregular shape, spiculated-border mass with a round calcification adjacent to it located in the upper outer quadrant of the left breast (arrow). Subsequently, a standard diagnostic mammogram in two views confirmed the similar findings (arrow). A core biopsy performed under ultrasound guidance revealed an invasive ductal carcinoma, which was found to be ER and PR positive and HER2 negative

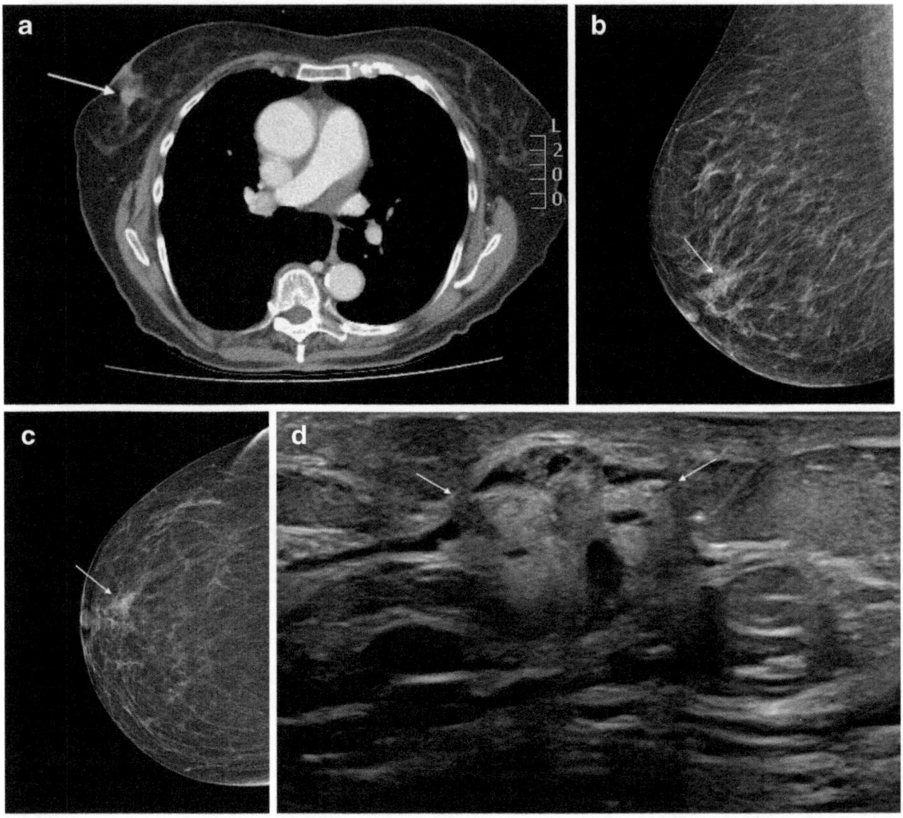

Fig. 1.3 Echogenic breast cancer. Axial CT chest with IV contrast (**a**), mammography MLO view (**b**), CC view (**c**), and grayscale ultrasound (**d**). Chest CT scan demonstrates an irregular shape, enhancing subcentimeter mass located in the retroareolar region of the right breast. In mammography, only a subtle focal asymmetry without any associated calcifications or architectural distortion is detected. In targeted ultrasound, corresponding to the CT scan findings, a heterogeneous echogenic solid mass is present in the same location. Classically, hyperechoic lesions on breast ultrasound are deemed likely benign; however, they might uncommonly be malignant. This mass underwent an ultrasound-guided biopsy with a malignant result, invasive carcinoma with lobular features, ER positive, PR positive, HER2 negative

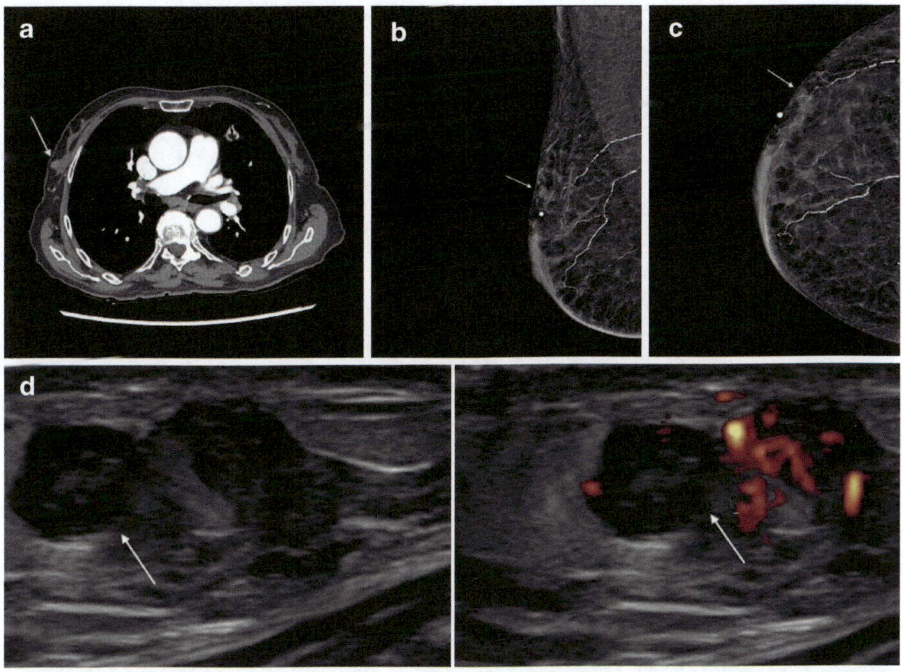

Fig. 1.4 Small superficial mass. Axial CT chest with IV contrast (**a**), mammography MLO view (**b**), and CC view (**c**), and grayscale ultrasound and color Doppler (**d**). Chest CT scan demonstrates a superficially located nodularity in the right lateral breast with very subtle enhancement (arrow). A standard diagnostic mammogram in two views confirmed a nodular focal asymmetry in the same location (arrow), which was also palpable by the patient and marked with a BB marker. In addition, the patient had a history of chronic renal failure with reported generalized edema. Breast skin thickening in the dependent part and significant vascular calcifications may reflect the history. In ultrasound, a corresponding vascular, solid, lobulated mass was detected, which underwent a core biopsy, yielding an invasive ductal carcinoma, which was found to be ER and PR positive, and HER2 negative

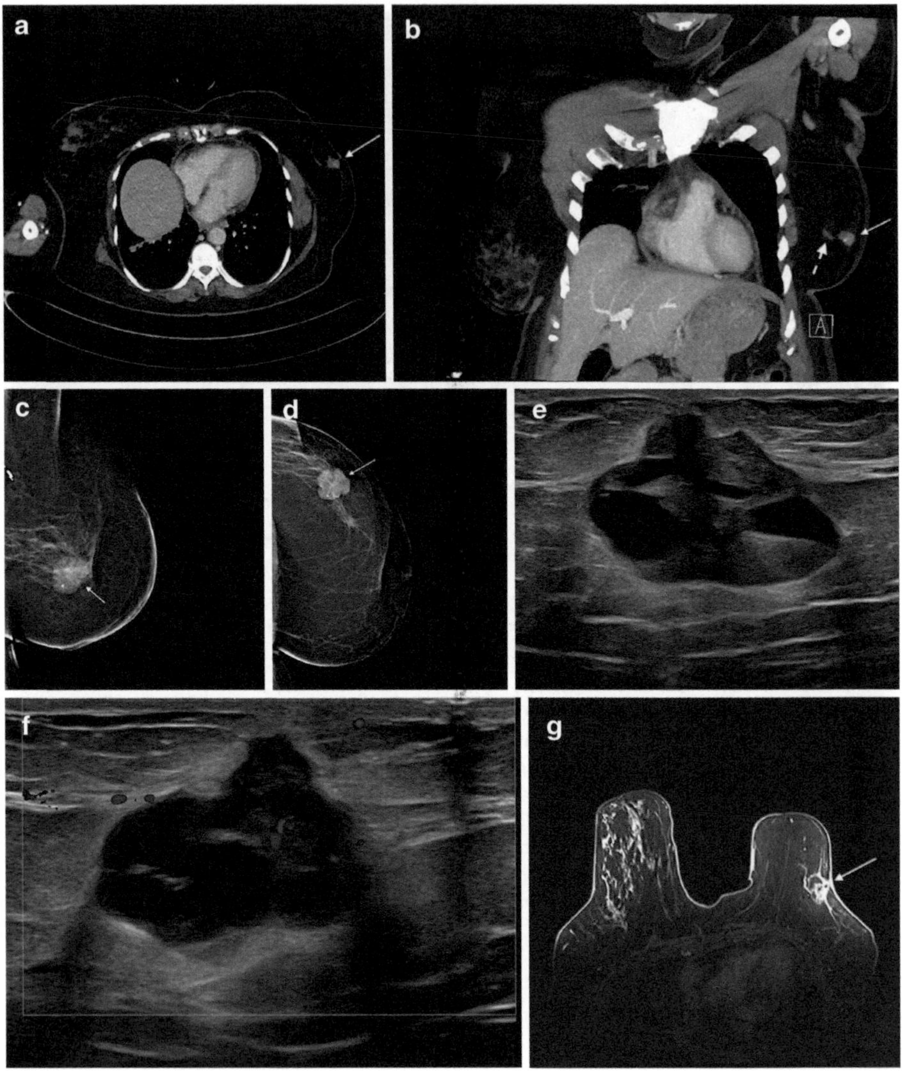

Fig. 1.5 Breast cancer in DIEP flap reconstruction. Axial CT chest with IV contrast (**a**), coronal reconstructed CT (**b**), mammography MLO view (**c**), CC view (**d**), grayscale ultrasound (**e**), color Doppler (**f**), and axial fat-saturated subtracted MRI (**g**) images of a patient with a history of left breast remote mastectomy and reconstruction DIEP flap. The chest CT scan reveals a fatty reconstructed breast with an irregular shape, heterogeneous-enhancing soft tissue mass within the lateral central breast, located superficially close to the skin, associated with a linear soft tissue density that is better visualized in the coronal view (dashed arrow). Mammography of the reconstructed breast confirmed the presence of the mass in the left lateral breast, and the mass appears more lobulated. The selected mammography image was obtained after biopsy and clip placement. A radiopaque clip is within the mass, and there are signs of hematoma surrounding the mass. In targeted ultrasound, a heterogeneous, solid-cystic, mildly vascular mass close to the skin was detected, which underwent an ultrasound-guided biopsy and yielded invasive ductal carcinoma, ER/PR negative and HER2 positive. MRI demonstrated a heterogeneous, avidly enhancing mass associated with linear non-mass enhancement anterior and posteriorly

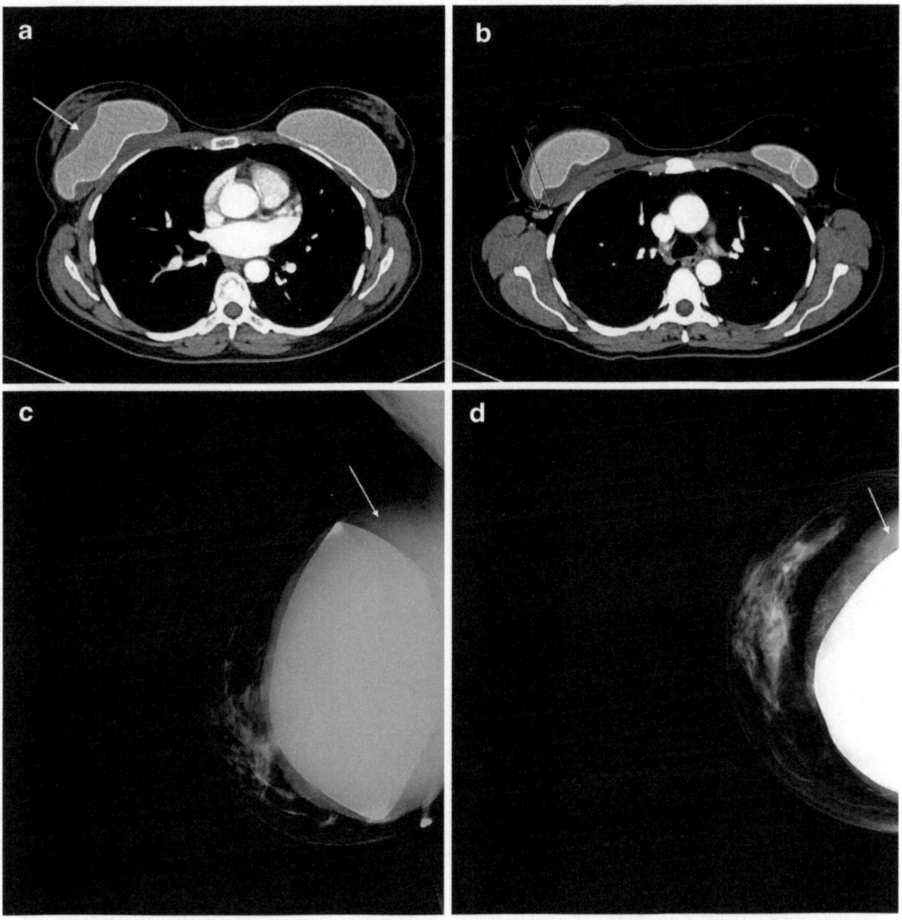

Fig. 1.6 Implant-associated anaplastic large cell lymphoma (ALCL). Axial CT chest with IV contrast (**a**, **b**), mammography MLO view (**c**), CC view (**d**), and grayscale ultrasound (**e**, **f**) of a patient with a history of bilateral remote textured silicone implants. Chest CT scan demonstrates right breast collapsed implant associated with significant peri-implant fluid contained within the fibrotic capsule (arrow in **a**). An enlarged enhancing node in the right axilla was also detected (arrow in **b**). Mammography indicates a right breast retroglandular deformed silicone implant with two distinct surrounding densities. The lower density corresponds to fluid surrounding the implant. Ultrasound confirmed the presence of substantial peri-implant fluid and an enlarged lymph node in the axilla. An ultrasound-guided fluid aspiration and core biopsy of the axillary node were performed, which ultimately yielded a diagnosis of implant-associated anaplastic large cell lymphoma (ALCL)

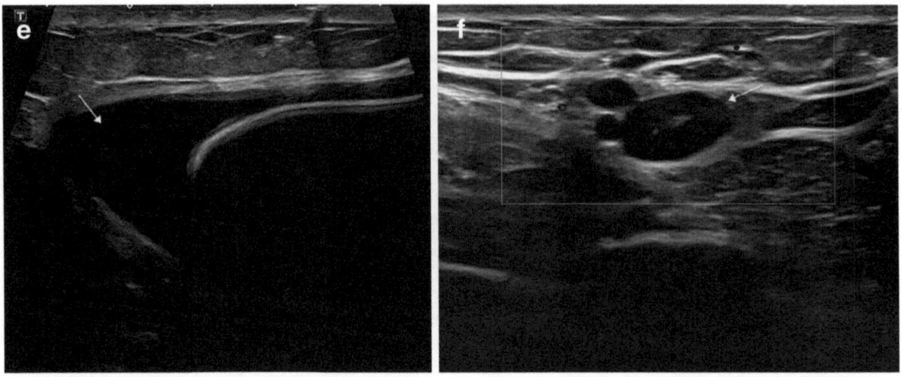

Fig. 1.6 (continued)

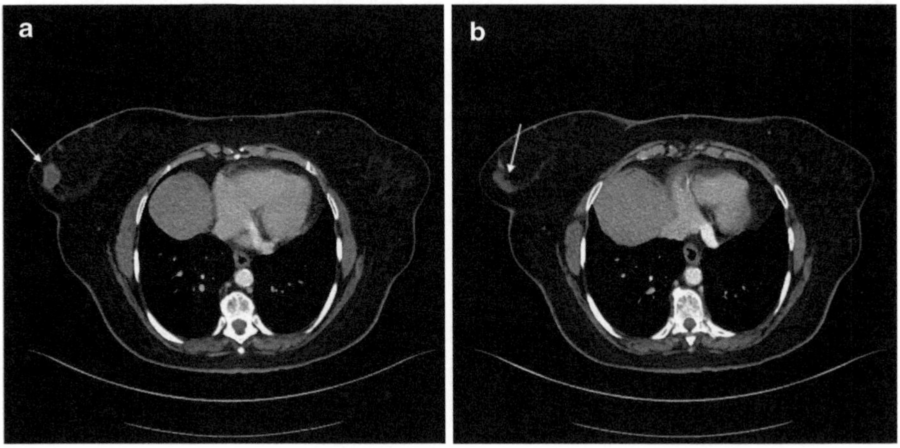

Fig. 1.7 Cancer with two components. Axial CT chest with IV contrast (**a**, **b**), mammography MLO view (**c**), CC view (**d**), and color Doppler ultrasound (**e**) images. Chest CT scan demonstrates an irregular mass with thick rim enhancement and central low density located in the right lateral central breast (arrow in **a**), associated with a linear component extending outside the mass posteriorly (arrow in **b**). Mammography indicates an irregular mass associated with an oblong asymmetry, which corresponds to the bilobed heterogeneous vascular solid mass in ultrasound at approximately 9:00. The mass underwent ultrasound-guided biopsy, and pathology came as invasive breast carcinoma with mucinous features and neuroendocrine differentiation, with ER, PR receptor positive and HER2 negative

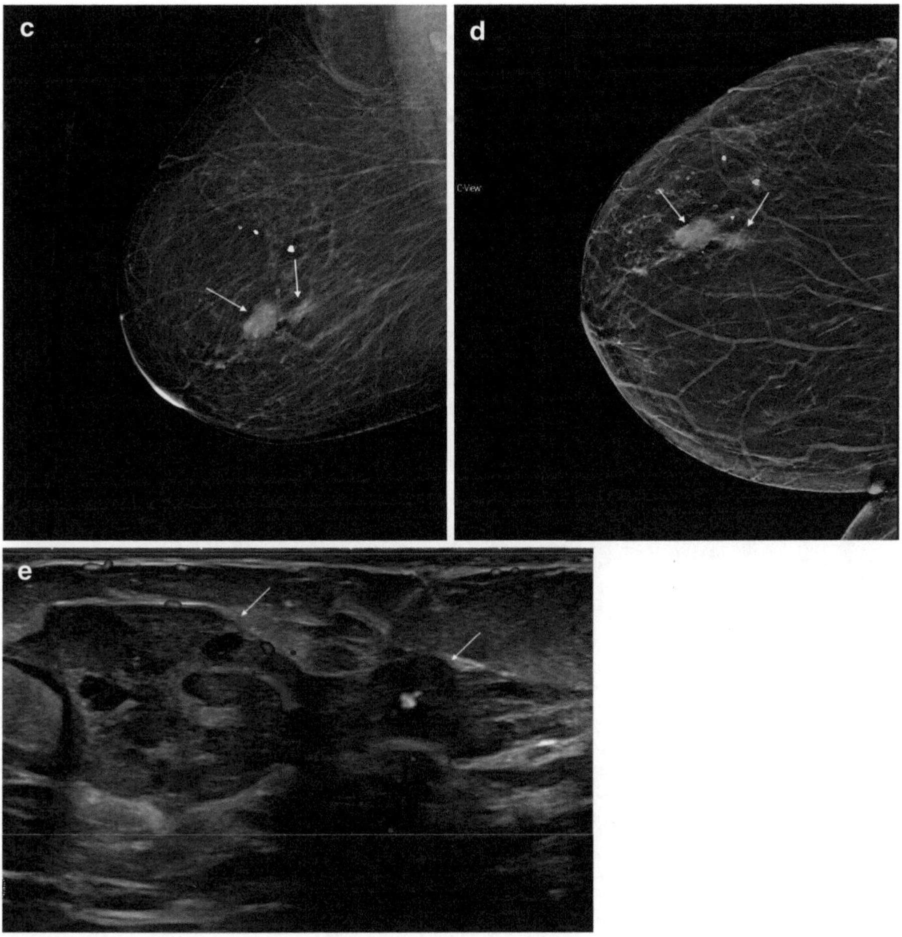

Fig. 1.7 (continued)

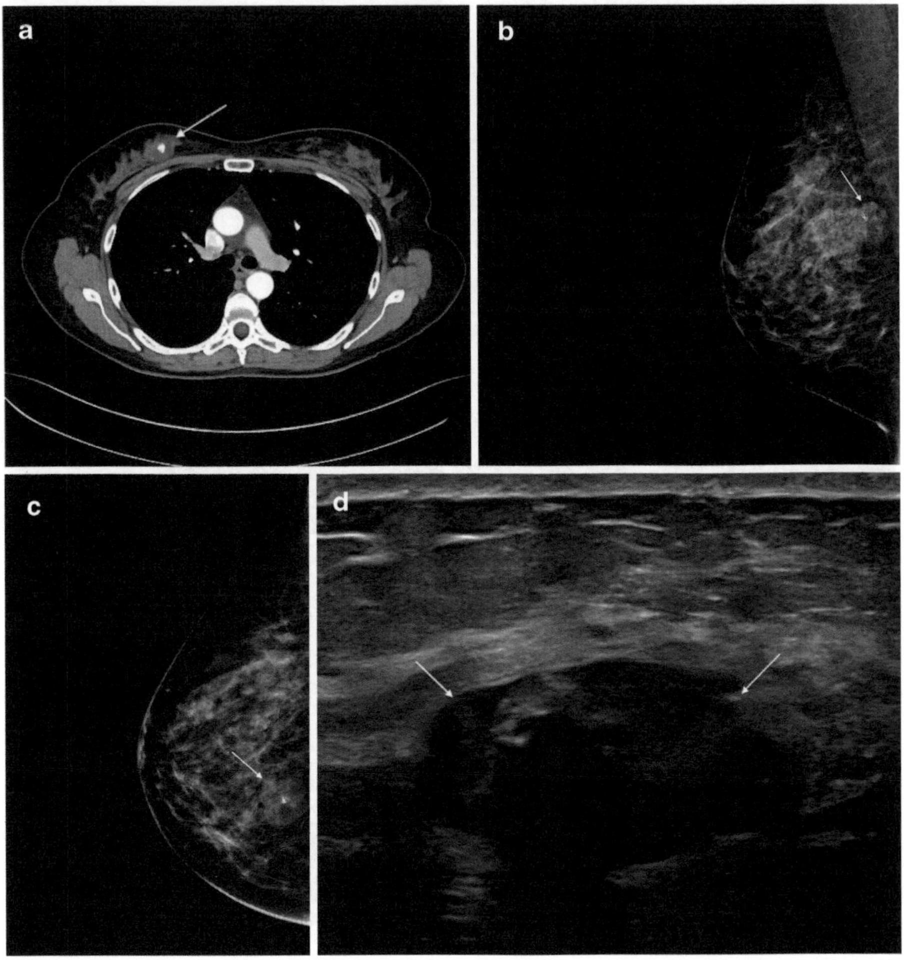

Fig. 1.8 Malignant phyllodes tumor. Axial CT chest with IV contrast (**a**), mammography MLO view (**b**), CC view (**c**), grayscale ultrasound (**d**), and color Doppler ultrasound (**e**) images. Chest CT scan demonstrates a soft tissue mass with slight enhancement associated with a macrocalcification in the right upper inner posterior breast. Mammography reveals a partially obscured, isodense mass with central calcification and dystrophic morphology. An ultrasound examination revealed a circumscribed, lobulated hypoechoic solid mass with internal bright echo and posterior shadowing, indicating the presence of calcifications. Additionally, an adjacent feeding vessel was observed. An ultrasound-guided biopsy yielded the rare diagnosis of malignant spindle-cell lesion with pleomorphic liposarcomatous differentiation and focal myxochondroid stroma, favoring malignant phyllodes tumor

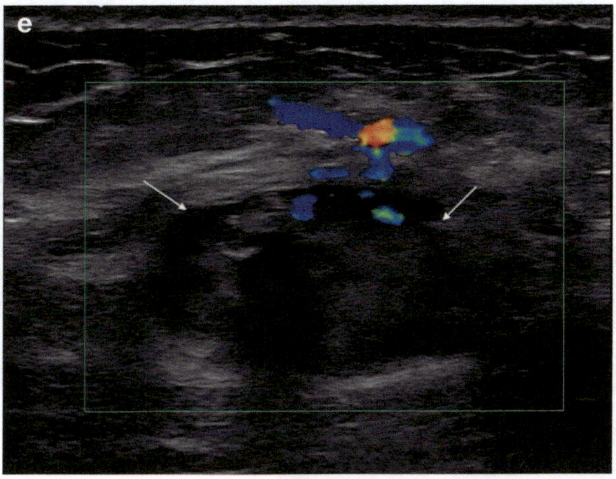

Fig. 1.8 (continued)

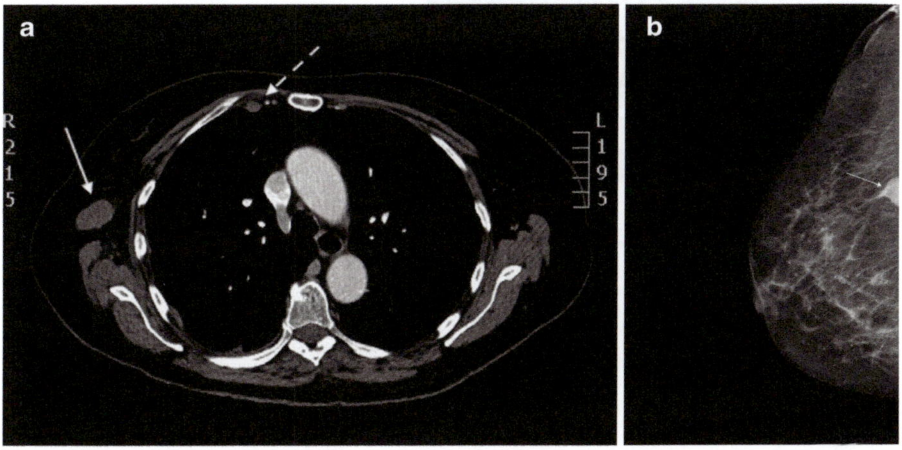

Fig. 1.9 Ovarian Müllerian tumor metastasis to breast. Axial CT chest with IV contrast (**a**), exaggerated CC view (**b**), grayscale ultrasound (**c**), color Doppler ultrasound (**d**), and axial CT abdomen with IV contrast (**e**) images. Chest CT scan demonstrates an oval soft tissue mass in upper outer right breast without significant enhancement in visual assessment (arrow) and enlarged right internal mammary lymph node (dashed arrow). The mammography indicated a partially included, posteriorly located, dense mass, which corresponds to a heterogeneous, hypoechoic, solid mass in ultrasound, with no significant flow in the color Doppler image. The ultrasound-guided biopsy resulted in a metastasis from her known malignant mixed Müllerian tumor of the ovary. Axial abdominal CT scan showed liver surface nodular metastasis (solid arrow) and abdominal ascites (dashed arrow)

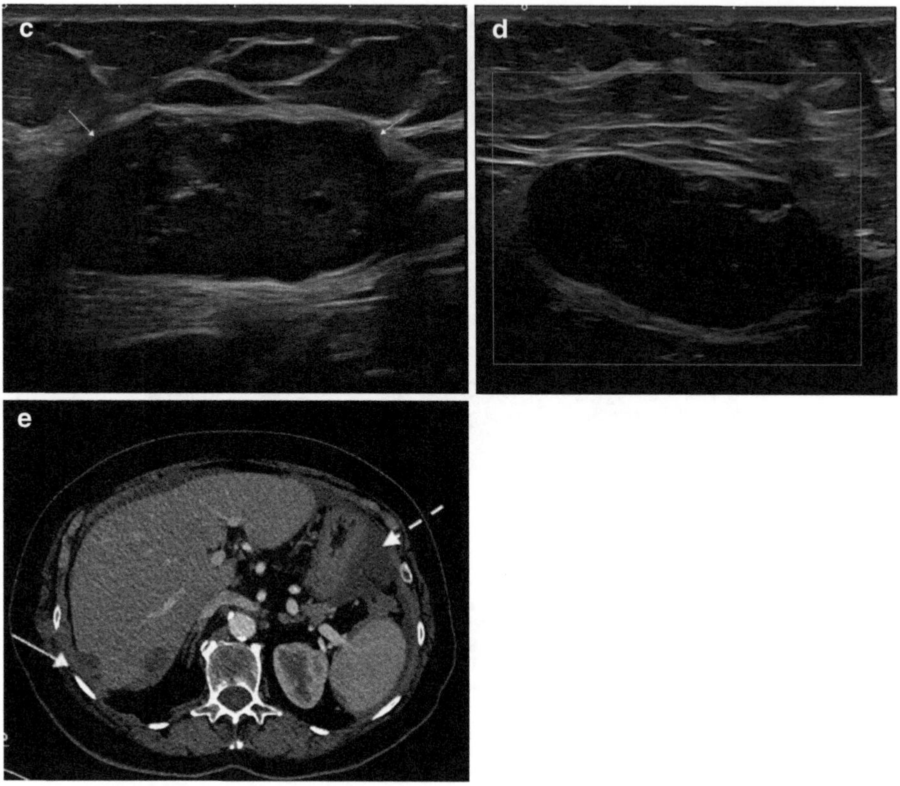

Fig. 1.9 (continued)

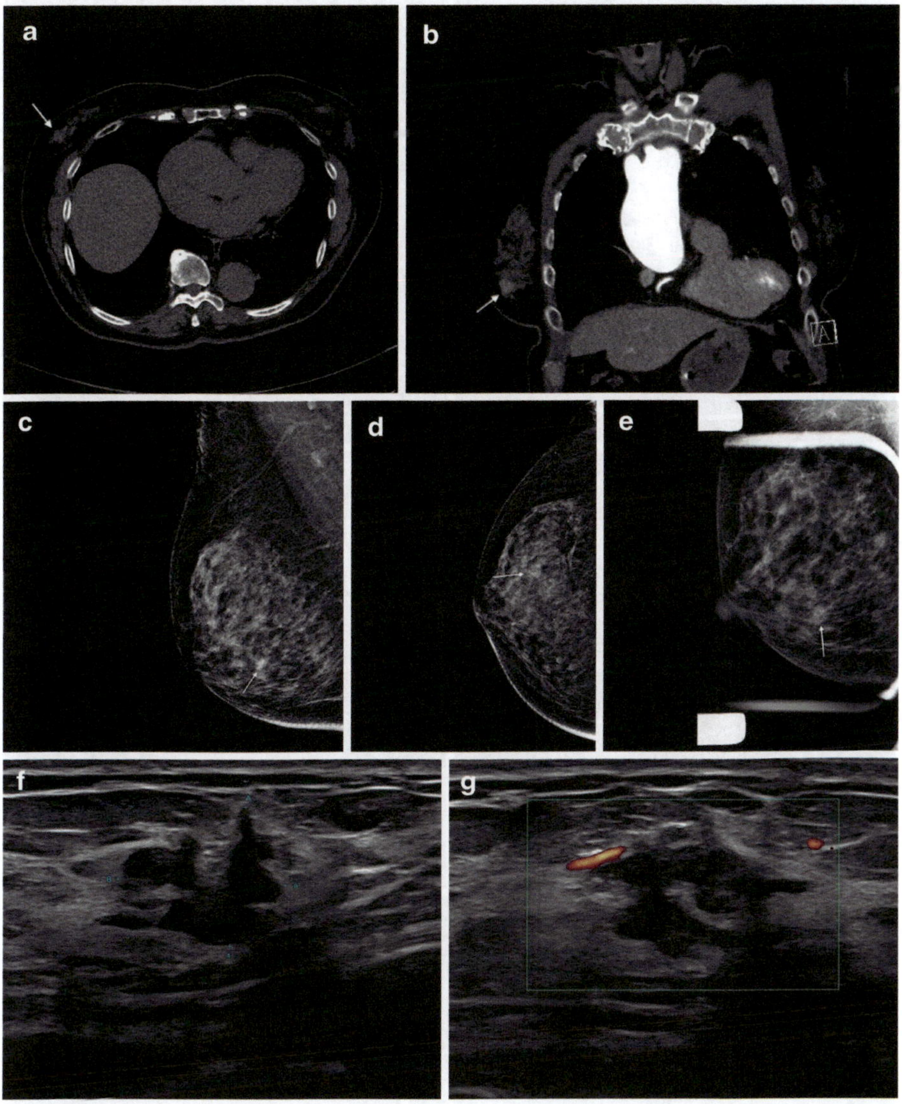

Fig. 1.10 Incidentally detected cancer in chest CT scan without contrast. Chest CT scan without IV contrast axial (**a**), with IV contrast coronal reconstruction (**b**), mammography MLO view (**c**), CC view (**d**), magnification view (**e**), grayscale ultrasound (**f**), and color Doppler (**g**). Chest CT images detected an incidental dense nodularity in the right lower outer breast, which enhances after contrast injection. Mammography revealed a focal asymmetry in the right lower outer breast, associated with some slightly pleomorphic microcalcifications, confirmed in magnification views. Ultrasound examination identified an irregularly shaped, hypoechoic solid mass with some peripheral vascularity and internal bright echoes, corresponding to calcifications in the mammogram. An ultrasound-guided biopsy confirmed the presence of invasive, non-special type (ductal) carcinoma with an in situ component, and the tumor was found to be ER positive, PR positive, and HER2 negative

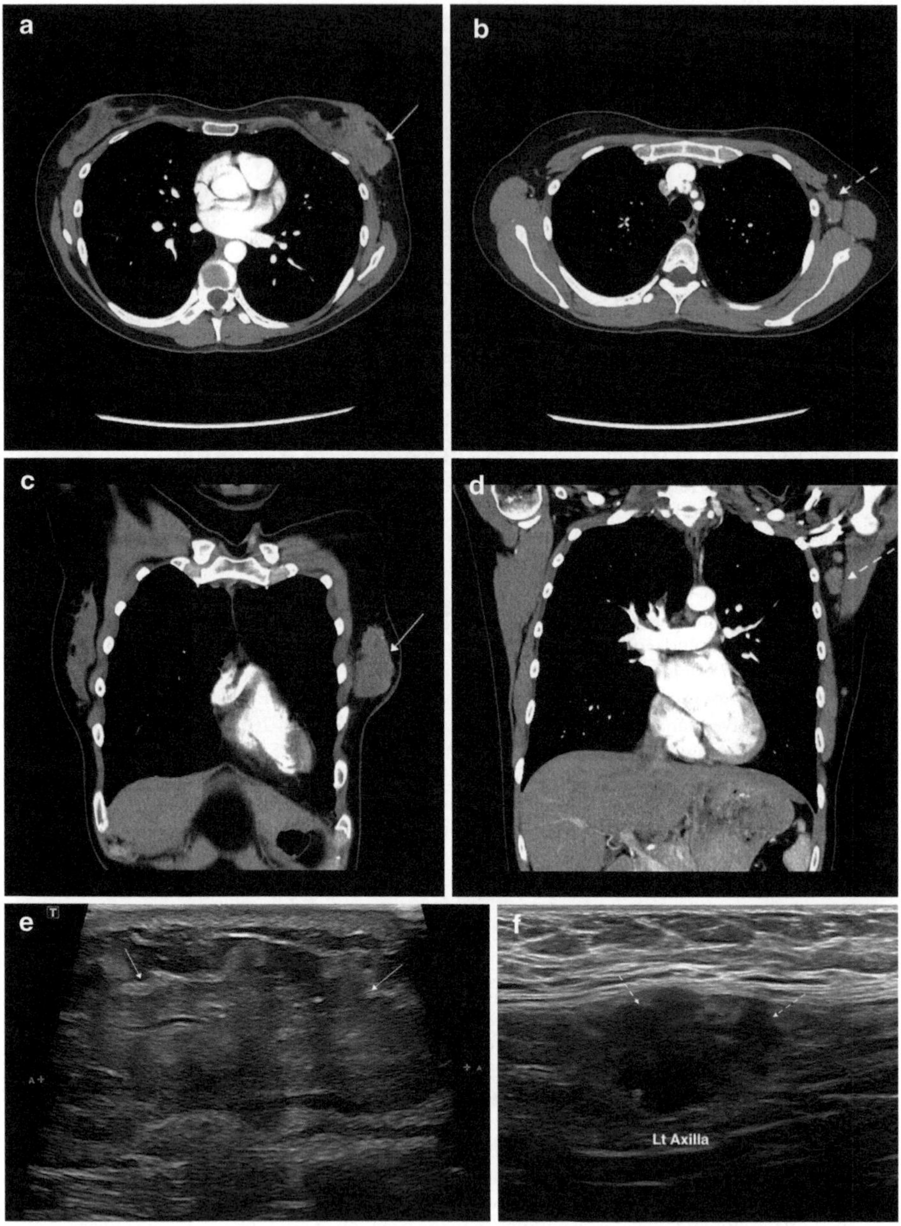

Fig. 1.11 Breast cancer with PET scan correlation. Axial CT chest with IV contrast (**a**, **b**), coronal chest CT scan with IV contrast (**c**, **d**), grayscale ultrasound (**e**, **f**), and PET scan (**g**, **h**). Chest CT scan demonstrates a large soft tissue mass with slight enhancement in the left lateral breast (arrow). There are at least two enlarged lymph nodes in the left axilla, level I (dashed arrow). Ultrasound also revealed a large, heterogeneous soft tissue mass corresponding to the chest CT findings, as well as enlarged axillary lymph nodes with an effaced hilum, which is highly suspicious for metastatic infiltration. The PET CT scan confirmed the same findings, with more axillary nodes showing increased uptake. Ultrasound-guided core needle biopsy of the breast and node yielded an invasive ductal carcinoma, which was found to be ER and PR positive, and HER2 negative

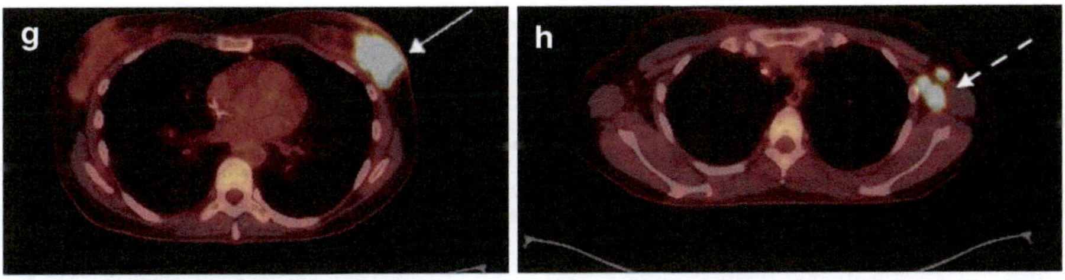

Fig. 1.11 (continued)

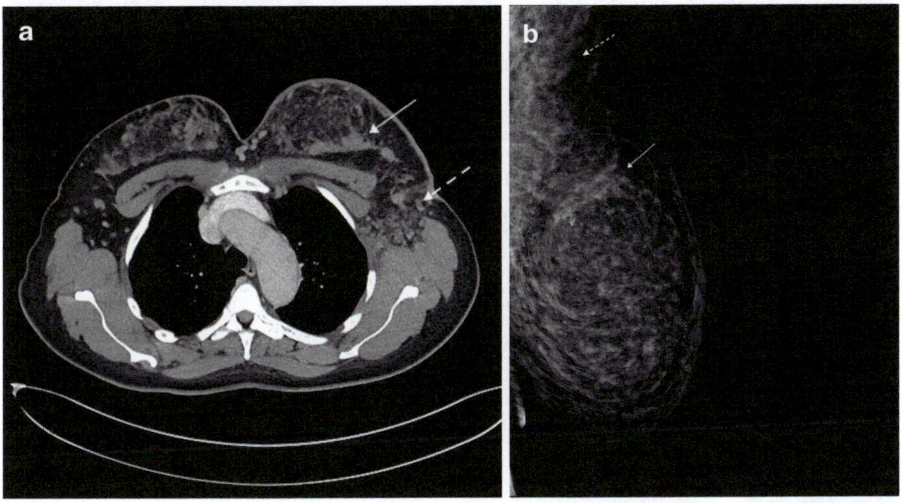

Fig. 1.12 Inflammatory breast cancer. Axial CT chest with IV contrast (**a**), mammography MLO view (**b**), grayscale ultrasound (**c, d**), and coronal orbital CT with contrast (**e**). Chest CT scan demonstrates left breast skin thickening, breast edema, upper breast irregular shape soft tissue mass (solid arrow) and infiltrative soft tissue in the axilla (dashed arrow). The left breast mediolateral-view mammogram showed the same findings, including significant skin thickening, extensive edema, upper breast mass (solid arrow), and axillary infiltrative soft tissue mass (dashed arrow). The ultrasound indicated a spiculated, irregular, hypoechoic solid mass with a posterior shadow corresponding to the upper breast mass in the CT scan and mammogram (arrow). Skin thickening and edema were also documented in ultrasound (**d**). The ultrasound-guided biopsy confirmed the diagnosis of inflammatory breast cancer. Patient reported significant vision loss, and a CT scan of the brain and orbits was performed (**e**), indicating soft tissue involvement in the right orbital area affecting the orbital muscles (arrows), which was also biopsied and confirmed as metastasis from breast cancer

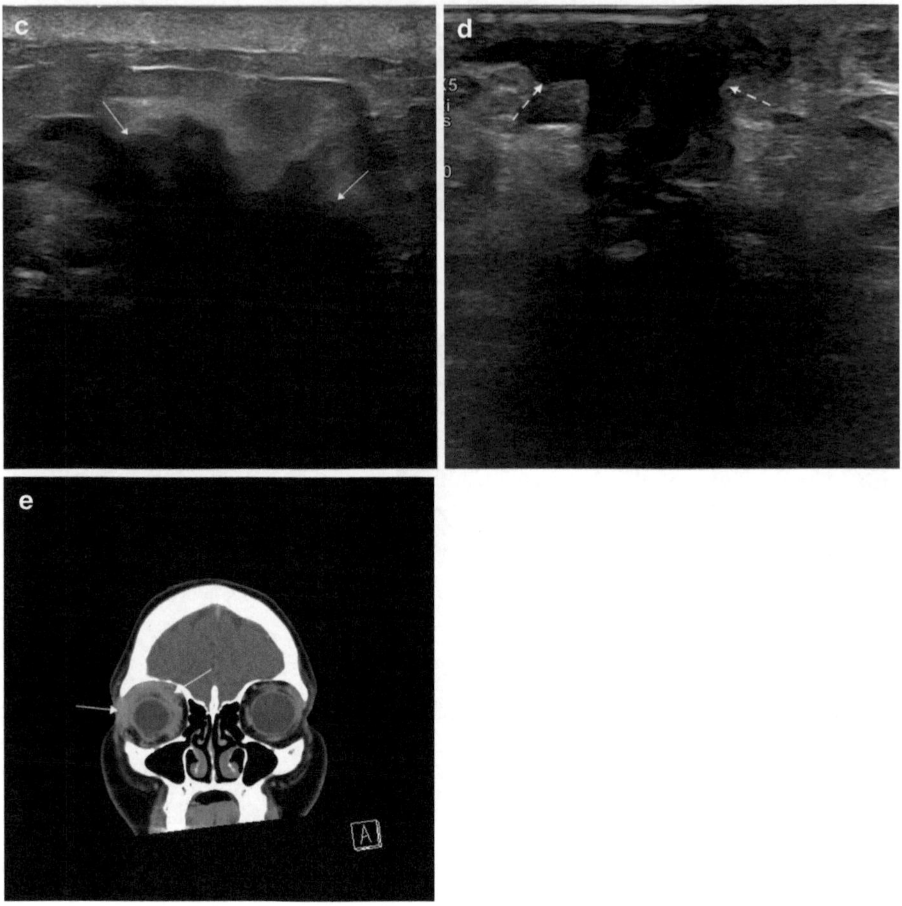

Fig. 1.12 (continued)

Fig. 1.13 Papillary breast carcinoma. Axial CT chest without IV contrast (**a**), coronal reconstructed CT chest without IV contrast (**b**), mammography MLO view (**c**), CC view (**d**), grayscale ultrasound (**e**), and color Doppler ultrasound (**f**). Chest CT scan demonstrates an irregular shape soft tissue mass with some internal lower-density components in the right upper slightly outer breast (arrow). Mammography with a BB marker corresponding to the patient's clinical concern of a lump, at the same location as the CT-detected mass, revealed a nodular asymmetry in the upper breast, which is not well visualized in the CC view. The ultrasound showed a hypoechoic, solid, vascular mass with internal cystic components. Ultrasound-guided core needle biopsy of this mass confirmed the diagnosis of papillary breast carcinoma

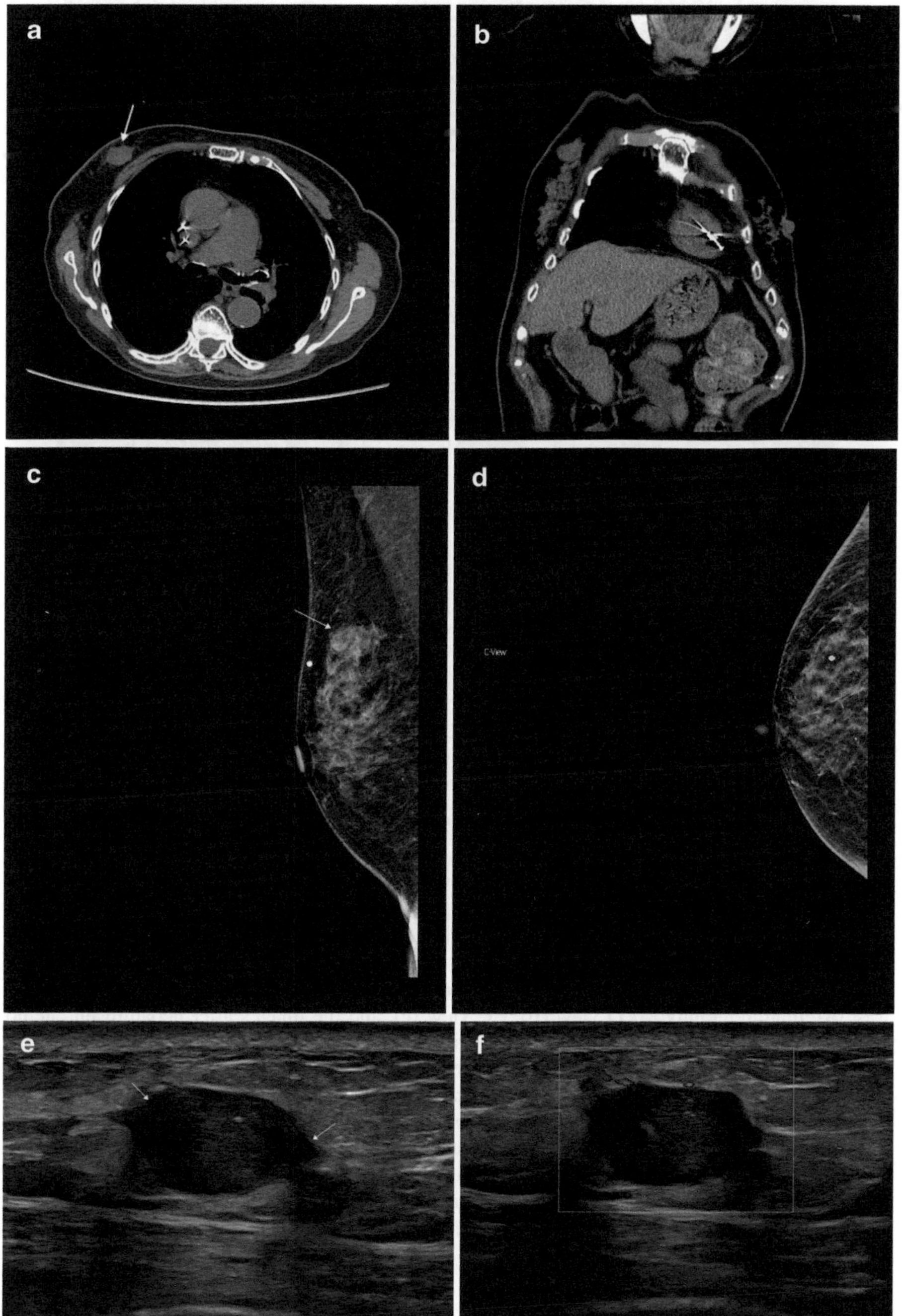
a
b
c
d
C-View
e
f

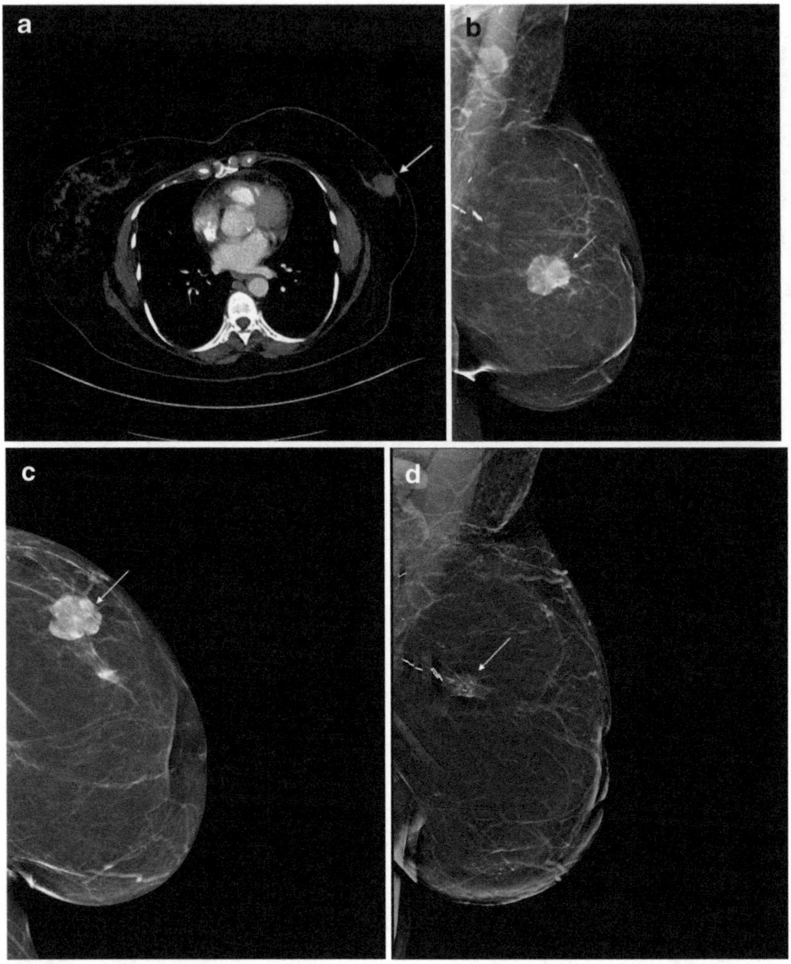

Fig. 1.14 Breast cancer before and after neoadjuvant chemotherapy. Axial CT chest with IV contrast (**a**), mammography MLO view (**b**), CC view (**c**), and the images after neoadjuvant chemotherapy axial CT chest with IV contrast (**d**), mammography MLO view (**e**), and CC view (**f**). In a patient with a remote history of left breast mastectomy and DIEP reconstruction, chest CT demonstrates an irregular shape, heterogeneous, enhancing mass in the left lateral central breast (arrow). Mammography of the fatty flap-reconstructed breast confirmed a lobulated mass at the same location, consistent with the CT findings. An ultrasound-guided biopsy confirmed the diagnosis of recurrent malignancy, specifically invasive ductal carcinoma, which is ER/PR negative and HER2 positive. Following this, the patient underwent neoadjuvant chemotherapy. The preoperative planning images show a partial response in both the chest CT scan and mammography

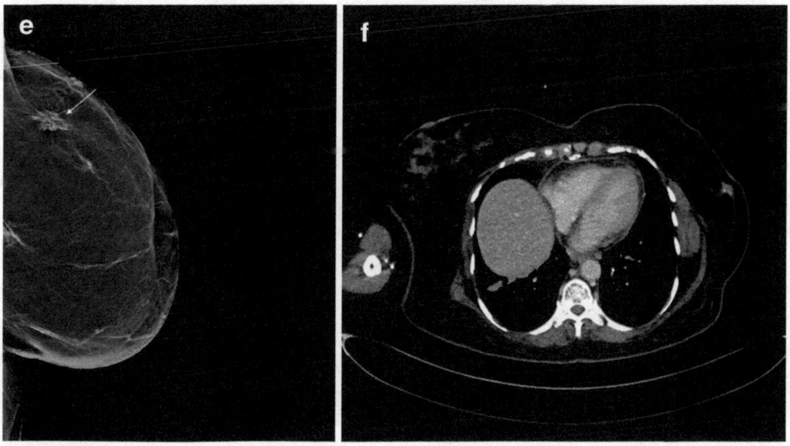

Fig. 1.14 (continued)

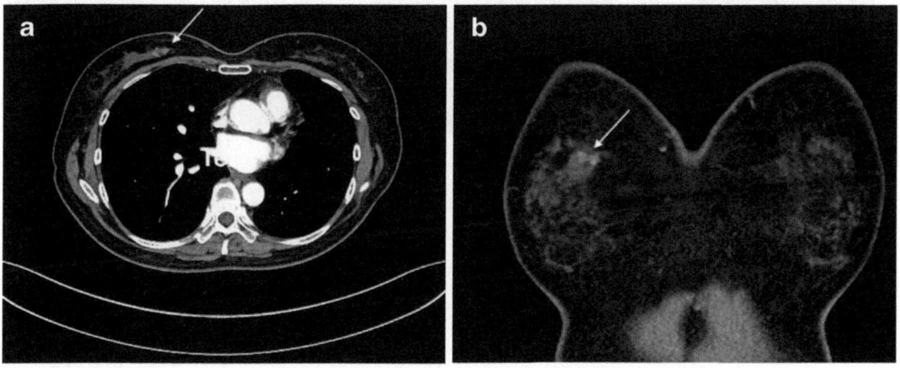

Fig. 1.15 Ductal carcinoma in situ (DCIS). Axial chest CT with IV contrast (**a**), coronal chest CT (**b**), axial chest CT (**c**), mammography MLO view (**d**), CC view (**e**), grayscale ultrasound (**f**), and color Doppler ultrasound (**g**). Chest CT demonstrates a non-mass enhancement in the right upper inner posterior breast (arrow). The lesion is not clearly seen in mammography, while a longstanding benign oval mass in the central breast is noted (dashed arrow). A targeted right upper inner breast ultrasound demonstrates an irregular hypervascular solid mass corresponding to CT scan findings. Ultrasound-guided biopsies yielded DCIS with apocrine features

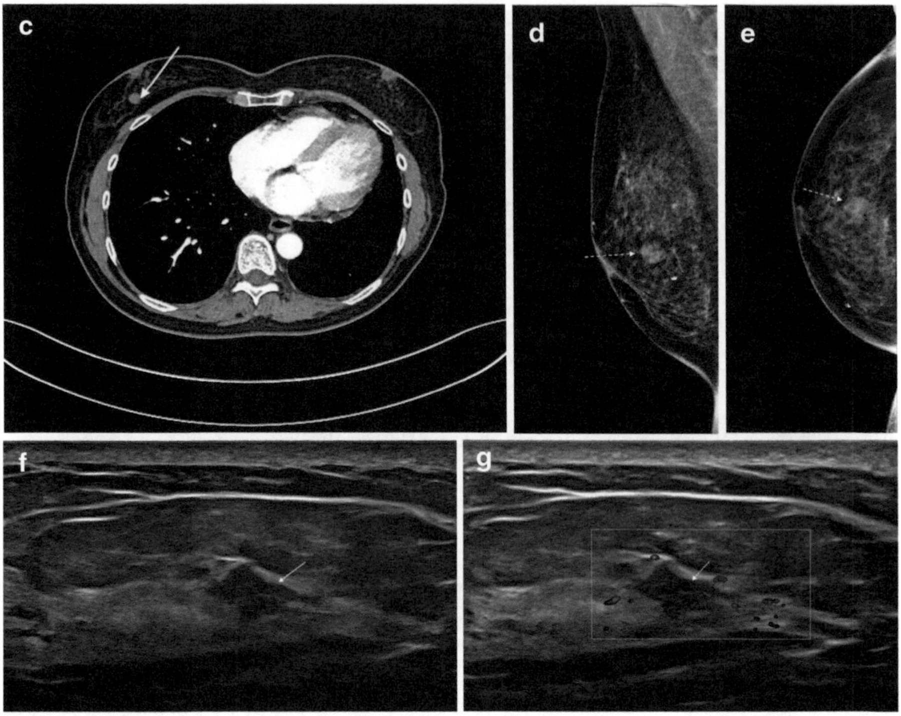

Fig. 1.15 (continued)

Fig. 1.16 Poorly differentiated carcinoma. Axial chest CT with IV contrast (**a**), coronal CT (**b**), MRI T1 sequence fat suppressed with contrast sagittal image (**c**), and MRI T1 sequence fat suppressed with contrast axial images (**d, e**). The chest CT revealed an infiltrative soft tissue mass (solid arrows) with indistinct borders in the right axilla, extending into the subpectoral, infraclavicular, and supraclavicular regions. There were also nodularities present in the upper breast (dashed arrows). The MRI images confirmed these findings, showing extensive non-mass enhancement in the upper outer breast that extended to the axillary regions (levels I, II, and III). Additionally, there was evidence of skin thickening and generalized breast edema. An ultrasound-guided examination of the lesion was performed, and the histological findings suggested poorly differentiated carcinoma. The immunohistochemical staining profile suggested a triple-negative (ER, PR, HER2 negative) breast cancer

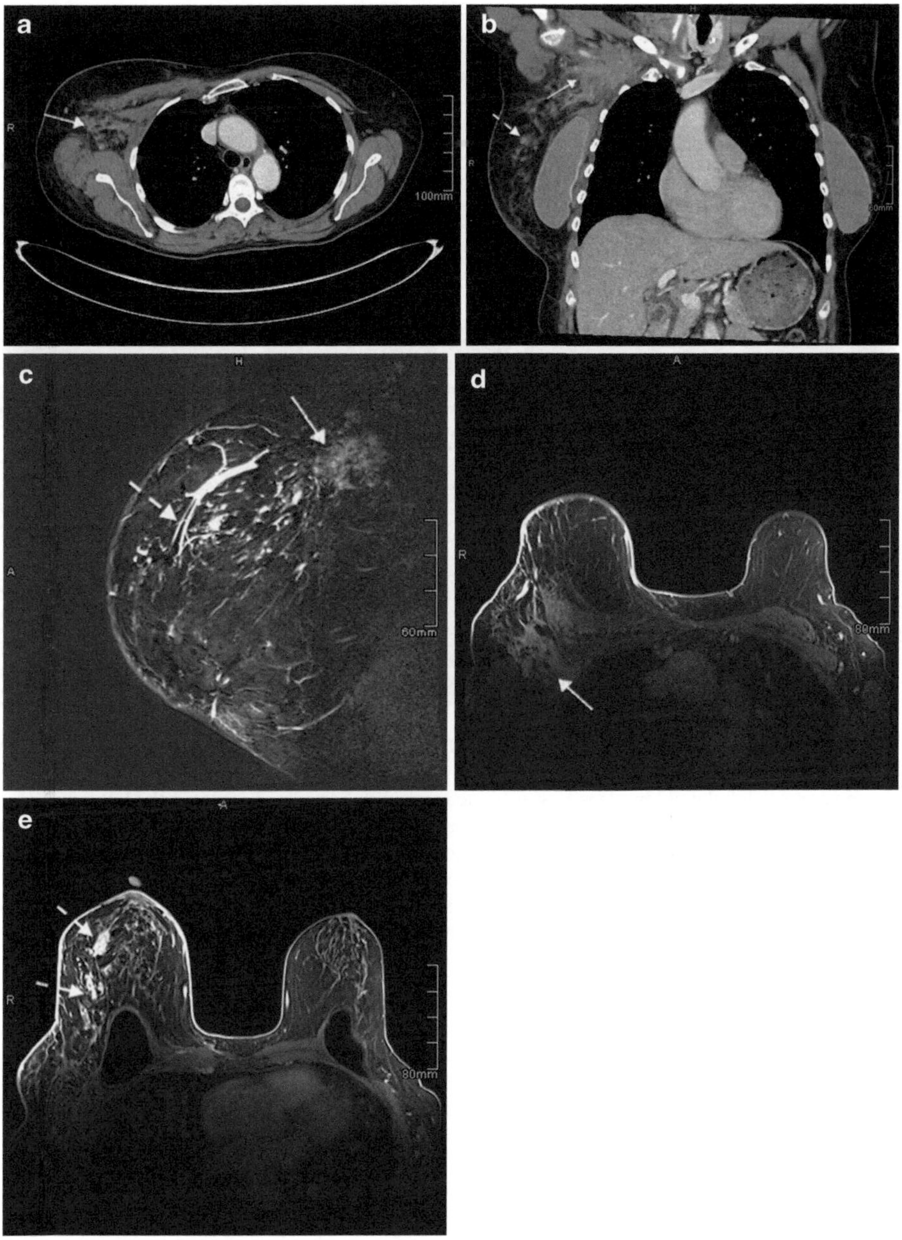
a
R
100mm
b
H
R
60mm
c
H
A
60mm
d
A
R
80mm
e
A
R
80mm

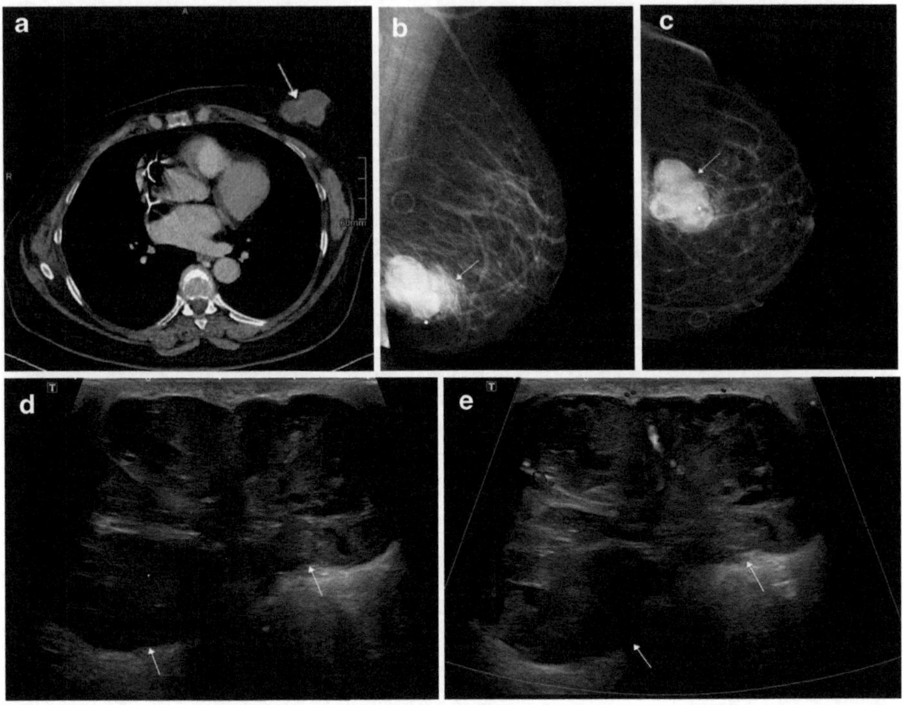

Fig. 1.17 Medullary breast carcinoma. Axial CT chest with IV contrast (**a**), mammography MLO view (**b**), CC view (**c**), grayscale ultrasound (**d**), and color Doppler ultrasound (**e**). Chest CT scan demonstrates a lobulated low-density soft tissue mass with rim enhancement in the left lower central breast (arrow). Mammography with a BB marker corresponding to the patient's clinical concern of a lump at the same location as the CT-detected mass revealed a dense, lobulated, large mass with no associated suspicious calcifications. The ultrasound showed a heterogeneous hypoechoic vascular solid with some internal cystic components. Ultrasound-guided core needle biopsy of this mass confirmed the diagnosis of triple-negative hormone receptor medullary breast cancer

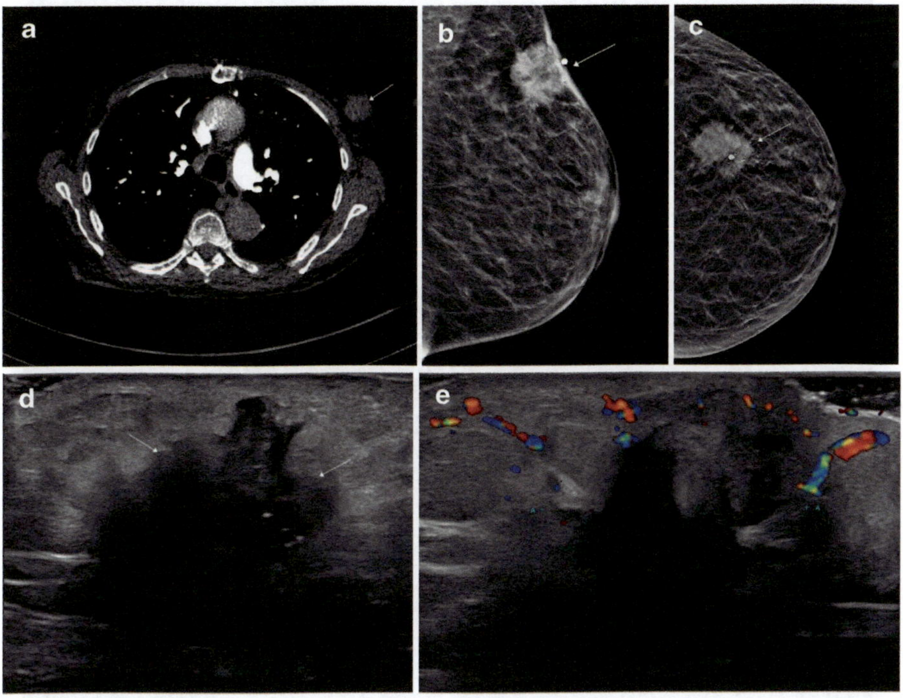

Fig. 1.18 Breast cancer with associated findings. Axial chest CT with IV contrast (**a**), mammography MLO view (**b**), CC view (**c**), grayscale ultrasound (**d**), and color Doppler (**e**). The chest CT scan reveals an irregular shape, spiculated border, heterogeneous, enhancing soft tissue mass in the left upper outer breast, with extension to the overlying skin, indicated by the arrow. Within the mass, there are tiny dense foci that may correspond to calcifications visible in the mammogram. In the mammography images, a BB marker is placed on the skin to identify the patient's area of concern. The mammogram shows an irregular shape mass with spiculated borders and some linear calcifications extending anteriorly and inferiorly, along with associated thickening of the overlying skin. The ultrasound reveals an irregularly shaped, spiculated solid mass that appears hypoechoic, with some dilated feeding vessels, increased peripheral echogenicity, and posterior shadowing, as seen in both grayscale and color Doppler imaging. A biopsy conducted using ultrasound guidance confirmed a diagnosis of invasive breast carcinoma

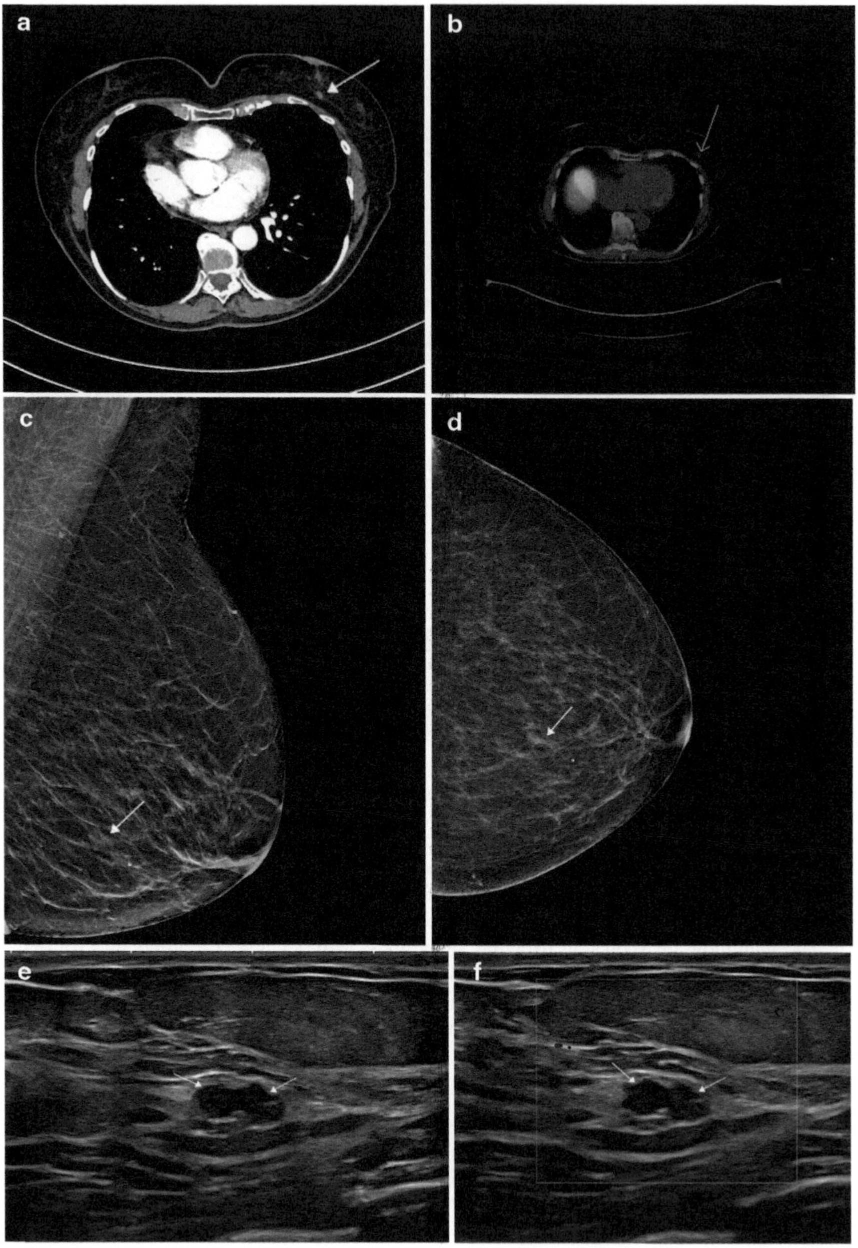

Fig. 1.19 Ductal carcinoma in situ (DCIS) in different modalities. Axial chest CT with IV contrast (**a**), PET CT scan (**b**), mammography MLO view (**c**), CC view (**d**), grayscale ultrasound (**e**), and color Doppler (**f**). The chest CT scan revealed a small, enhancing, oval-shaped mass in the left lower central breast. In the PET CT scan, conducted as part of the staging for her lung cancer, the same mass showed increased uptake. Mammography findings indicated a subtle focal asymmetry that corresponded to the CT scan results. Grayscale and color Doppler ultrasound identified an irregular-shaped, hypoechoic, hypovascular solid mass. A biopsy was performed under ultrasound guidance, which confirmed a diagnosis of ductal carcinoma in situ (DCIS)

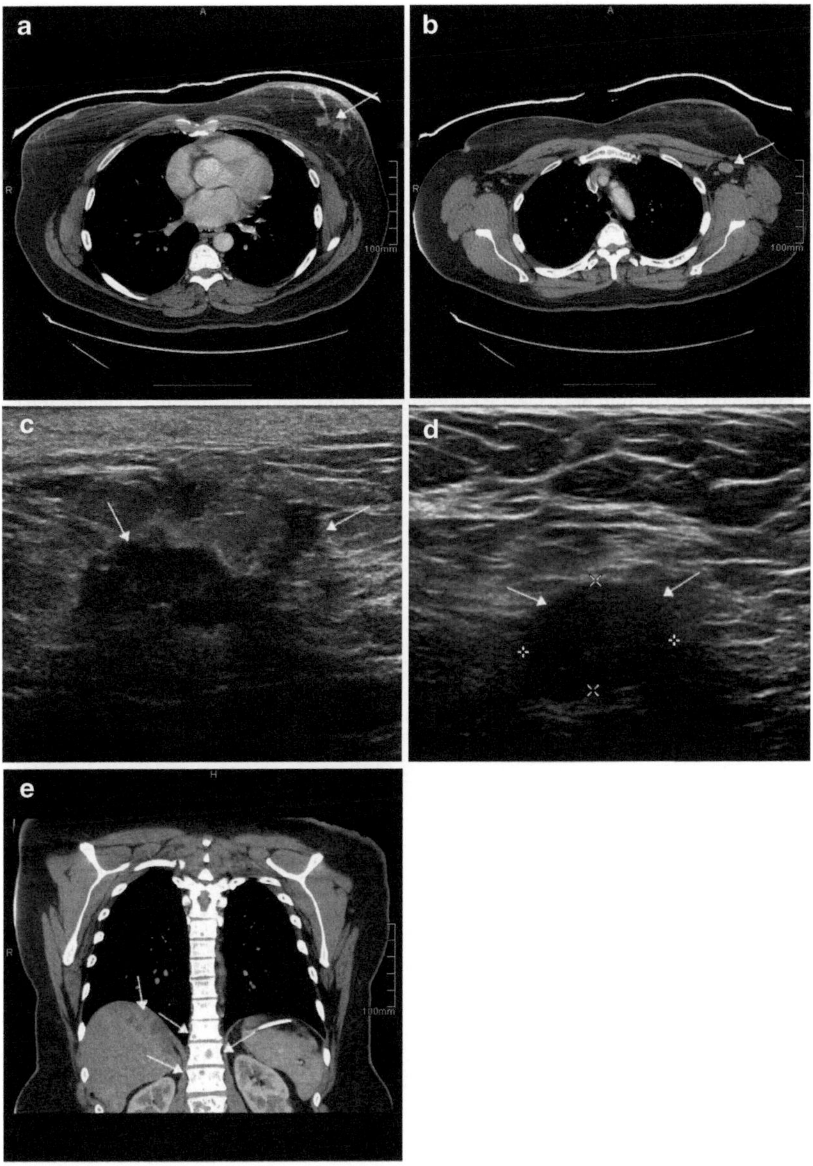

Fig. 1.20 One-stop shopping. Axial chest CT with IV contrast (**a, b**), grayscale breast ultrasound (**c**), grayscale axilla (**d**), and coronal chest CT scan (**e**). The chest CT revealed two interconnected, irregular shape masses with spiculated borders in the left lateral breast (indicated by the arrow in **a**), along with associated skin thickening. Additionally, a prominent lymph node in level I of the left axilla was detected (arrow in **b**). The ultrasound findings confirmed the presence of the two interconnected, irregular hypoechoic masses, which were associated with surrounding breast edema and skin thickening. The ultrasound also identified an enlarged level I lymph node in the left axilla, exhibiting increased cortical thickness and an effaced hilum. A biopsy of the larger mass in the breast confirmed a diagnosis of invasive breast carcinoma, and ultrasound-guided sampling of the left axillary lymph node was positive for malignancy. Further examination of the CT scan images (**e**) revealed multiple vertebral bone lesions and a heterogeneously enhancing mass at the liver dome (arrows), suggestive of metastasis

References

1. Desperito E, Schwartz L, Capaccione KM, Collins BT, Jamabawalikar S, Peng B, Patrizio R, Salvatore MM. Chest CT for breast cancer diagnosis. Life (Basel). 2022;12(11):1699. https://doi.org/10.3390/life12111699. PMID: 36362854; PMCID: PMC9695285
2. Park J, Kim C, Cha YK, Chung MJ. Missed and detected incidental breast cancers on contrast enhanced chest CT: detection rates and CT features. Diagnostics (Basel). 2023;13(9):1522. https://doi.org/10.3390/diagnostics13091522. PMID: 37174913; PMCID: PMC10177537
3. Choi YJ, Kim TH, Cha YJ, Son EJ, Gweon HM, Park CH. Incidental breast lesions on chest Ct: clinical significance and differential features requiring referral. J Korean Soc Radiol. 2018;79:303–10.
4. Harish MG, Konda SD, MacMahon H, Newstead GM. Breast lesions incidentally detected with Ct: what the general radiologist needs to know. Radiographics. 2007;27(Suppl. S1):S37–51.
5. Bach AG, Abbas J, Jasaabuu C, Schramm D, Wienke A, Surov A. Comparison between incidental malignant and benign breast lesions detected by computed tomography: a systematic review. J Med Imaging Radiat Oncol. 2013;57(5):529–33. https://doi.org/10.1111/1754-9485.12046. Epub 2013 Mar 26. PMID: 24119265

Chapter 2
Chest CT Appearance of Benign Breast Lesions

While CT scans are not commonly used for breast imaging, they can incidentally detect breast lesions, making it crucial for radiologists to characterize these findings accurately. According to the literature, most incidental breast lesions found on chest CT scans are benign [1].

Differentiating benign from malignant lesions in chest CT avoids unnecessary patient recall and additional imaging workup. Normal breast glandular tissue could appear as a pseudomass on a chest CT scan and cause unnecessary recalls and patient anxiety, which is more common in dense breasts. Compared with the contralateral breast, the previous chest CT scan and the available prior patient's dedicated breast imaging, especially mammography, prevent this misdiagnosis.

CT features, including shape, margin, and attenuation ratio, were significantly different between malignant and benign lesions [1]. None of the features alone could differentiate between benign and malignant lesions; however, the combination of findings is more diagnostic. Benign breast lesions can often be identified on chest CT scans by recognizing specific characteristics, such as an oval shape and well-circumscribed margins. In contrast, malignant lesions typically have irregular shapes and angulated or spiculated margins [2, 3].

The presence of enhancement alone does not always suggest a malignant tumor. Benign lesions usually show no enhancement, minimal enhancement, or homogeneous delayed enhancement, whereas malignant lesions may exhibit early rim enhancement or heterogeneous enhancement [4]. Chest CT is obtained for indications other than breast pathologies, and protocols are not optimized for breast imaging; therefore, variation in contrast medium administration and scan time is common. It has been suggested that the attenuation of breast lesions be compared with that of the ipsilateral trapezius muscle and reported as a ratio to correct for the diversity of enhancement protocols [1].

While not definitive, larger lesions and calcifications are associated with malignant conditions. However, these features alone are not reliable for distinguishing benign from malignant lesions [5].

A. Alikhassi, *Atlas of Breast Lesions on Chest Computed Tomography*,
https://doi.org/10.1007/978-3-032-22791-1_2

Fat-containing lesions, such as hamartomas and dystrophic or popcorn calcifications, are suggestive of benign etiologies [6]. The most common breast lesions are cysts, which typically appear as circumscribed or partially circumscribed non-enhancing masses with a Hounsfield unit less than 20 [7]. Fibroadenomas (FAs) are among the most common types of breast solid masses. They can be incidentally discovered during a chest CT scan or identified when the patient's history is retrieved [8].

To differentiate benign from malignant breast lesions on a chest CT scan, careful assessment of margins, shape, enhancement, and the presence of associated findings, such as skin thickening, calcifications, or axillary lymphadenopathy, is recommended. Comparing with previous images is critical.

Figures 2.1, 2.2, 2.3, 2.4, 2.5, 2.6, 2.7, 2.8, 2.9, 2.10, 2.11, 2.12, 2.13, 2.14, 2.15, 2.16, 2.17, 2.18, 2.19, 2.20 illustrate the detection of benign breast lesions in chest CT scans.

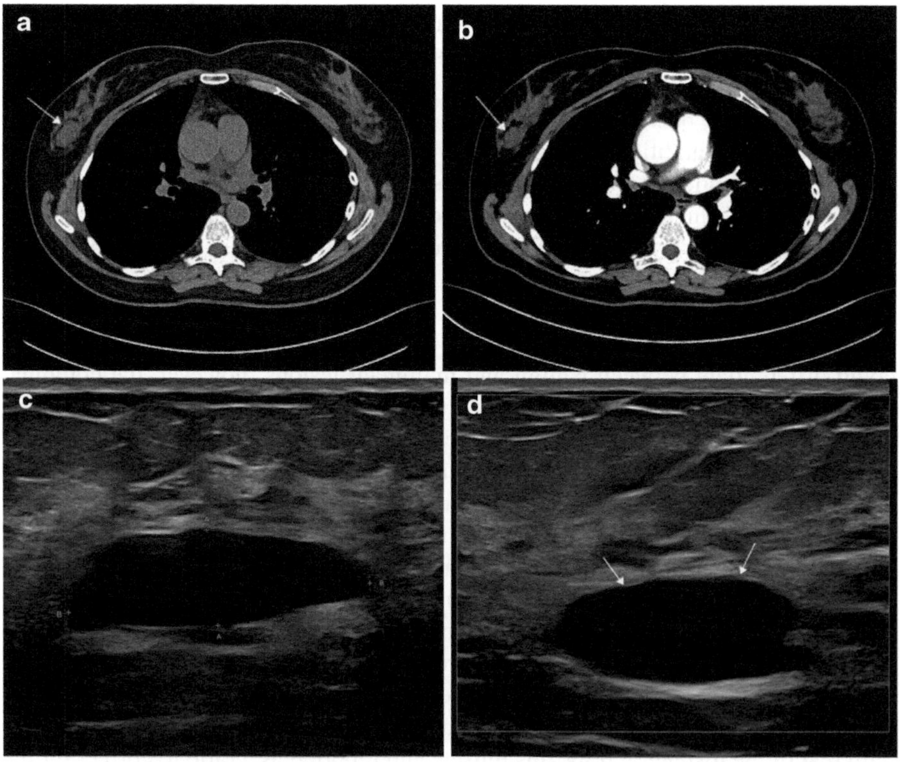

Fig. 2.1 Breast benign cyst. Axial chest CT scan without IV contrast (**a**), axial chest CT with IV contrast (**b**), grayscale ultrasound (**c**), and color Doppler ultrasound image (**d**). The chest CT image demonstrates an oval, circumscribed, low-density mass with a Hounsfield unit of less than 20 (arrow) within the right lateral posterior breast. After contrast injection, no significant change in the mass's density is observed. Ultrasound confirmed the presence of an oval, circumscribed, anechoic mass with posterior through transmission without color flow on Doppler, typical of a benign cyst

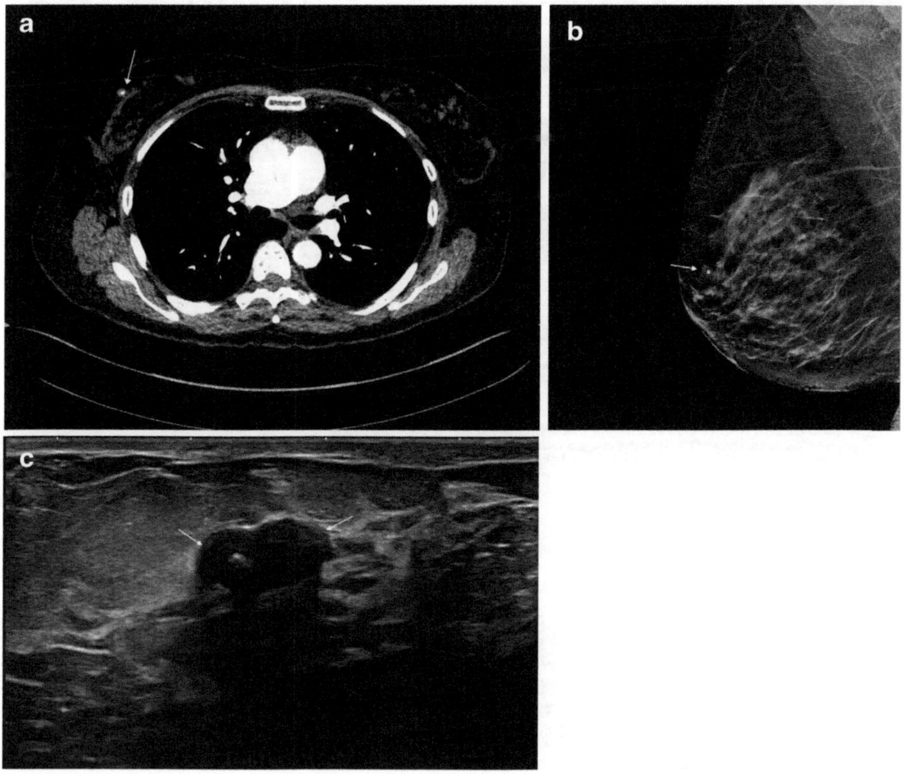

Fig. 2.2 Degenerated Fibroadenoma. Axial Chest CT scan with IV contrast (**a**), mammography MLO view (**b**), and grayscale ultrasound (**c**). Chest CT image demonstrates a circumscribed oval mass associated with a punctate calcification within the right upper breast (arrow). Mammography confirmed the same findings. A review of her older mammograms showed that the mass had been stable for more than 2 years. The ultrasound examination showed an oval, homogeneous, avascular, hypoechoic solid mass with a bright echo corresponding to the calcification on the mammogram. The findings suggest that the mass is a benign, degenerated fibroadenoma. Patient will continue routine screening mammogram

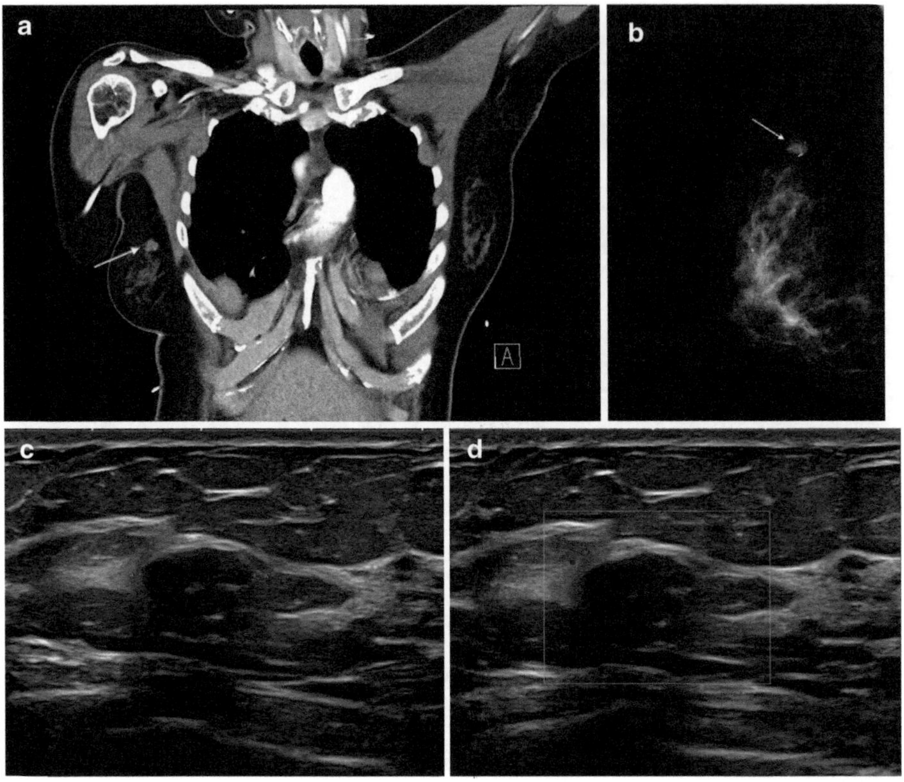

Fig. 2.3 Fibroadenoma. Coronal reconstructed chest CT scan with IV contrast (**a**), mammography MLO view (**b**), grayscale ultrasound (**c**), and color Doppler ultrasound (**d**). Chest CT image demonstrates a circumscribed lobulated soft tissue mass associated with punctate calcifications within the right upper breast (arrow). Mammography confirmed an oval, circumscribed soft tissue mass associated with some round and punctate calcifications (arrow). The mass appears homogeneous and hypoechoic on the ultrasound, with low vascularity in color Doppler. The patient had a remote biopsy of the same mass, which yielded benign fibroadenoma results

Fig. 2.4 Breast hematoma with active contrast blush. Axial chest CT scan with IV contrast (**a**), mammography MLO view (**b**), mammography CC view (**c**), focal compression view (**d**), grayscale ultrasound (**e**), and color Doppler ultrasound (**f**). Chest CT scan of a woman in a car accident demonstrates a large, dense, soft tissue mass in her right breast, suggestive of a hematoma (solid arrow), consistent with the clinical examination. Additionally, some blush of high attenuation contrast was noted in the superior aspect of the hematoma, indicating active arterial extravasation (dashed arrow). A few months after her discharge from the hospital, the patient expressed concern about a palpable mass remaining in her right breast. The mammograms revealed a band-shaped focal asymmetry (arrow) in the upper outer quadrant of the right breast, accompanied by dystrophic calcifications. An ultrasound showed a band-shaped, heterogeneous, hypoechoic lesion with posterior shadowing and minimal flow on color Doppler within the upper outer breast. The patient requested an ultrasound-guided biopsy of the palpable mass, which yielded scar tissue and fat necrosis with associated calcifications

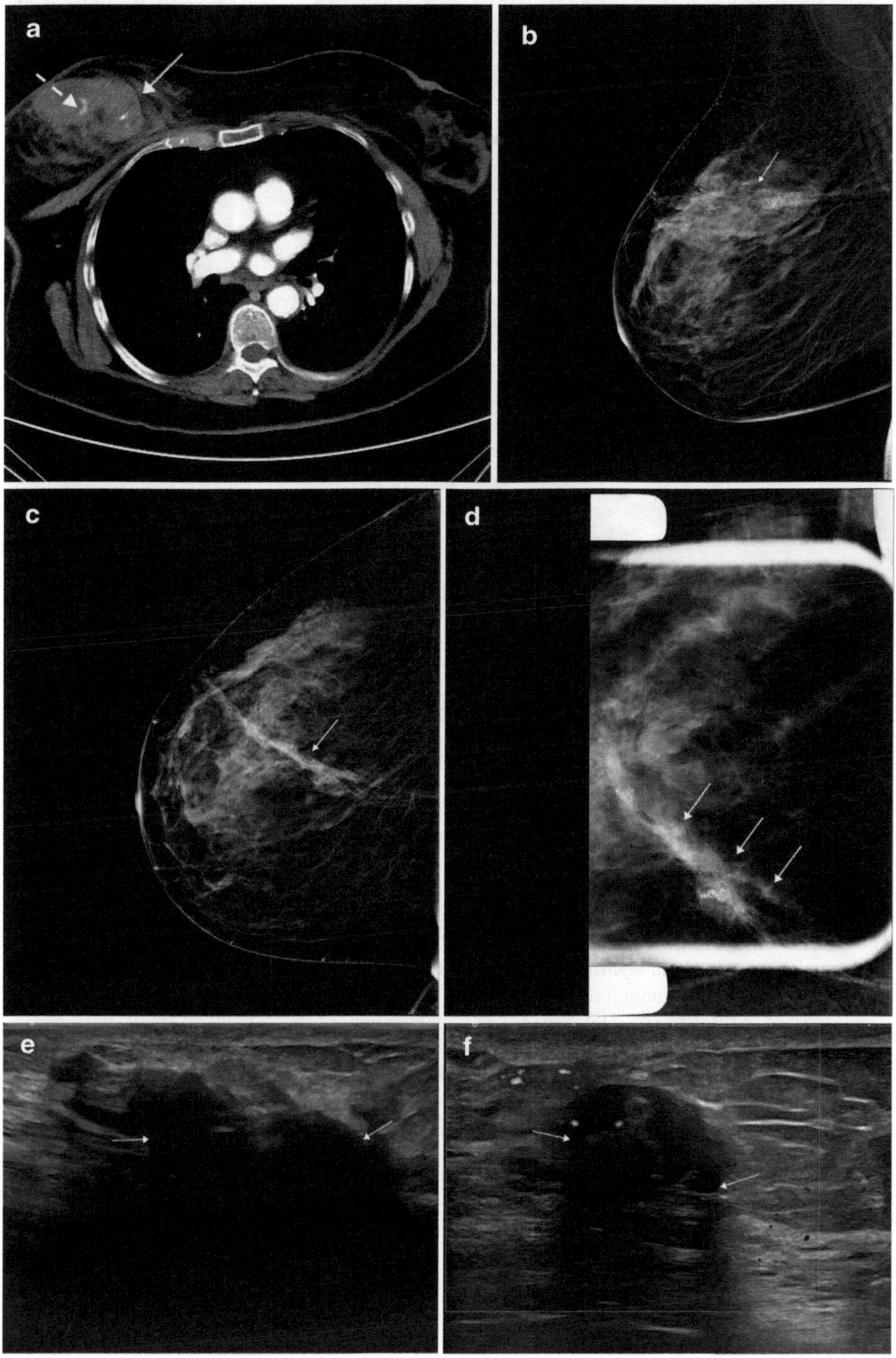
a
b
c
d
e
f

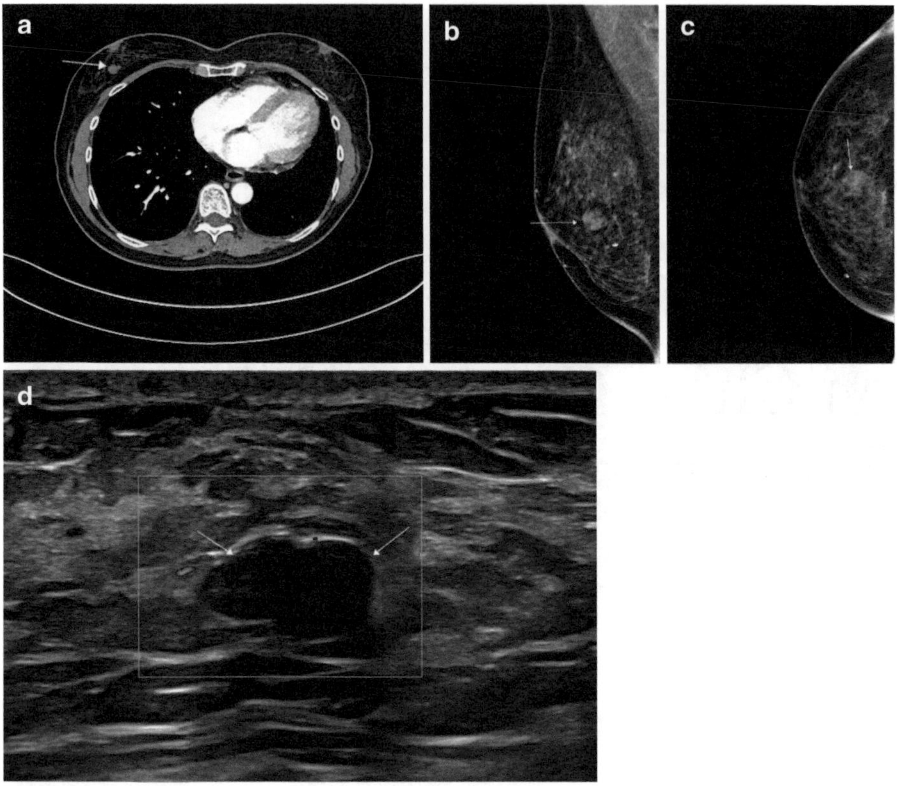

Fig. 2.5 Probably benign mass. Axial chest CT scan with IV contrast (**a**), mammography MLO view (**b**), CC view (**c**), and color Doppler ultrasound (**d**). Chest CT image demonstrates a circumscribed, lobulated, low-attenuating soft tissue mass within the right central middle third of the breast (arrow). Mammography shows a partially obscured oval isodense mass with no associated calcifications. The mass appears homogeneous, hypoechoic, and hypovascular on the ultrasound. The mass was reported as probably benign (BI-RADS 3), and a short-term follow-up ultrasound was suggested, with no change in follow-up, which confirmed benign

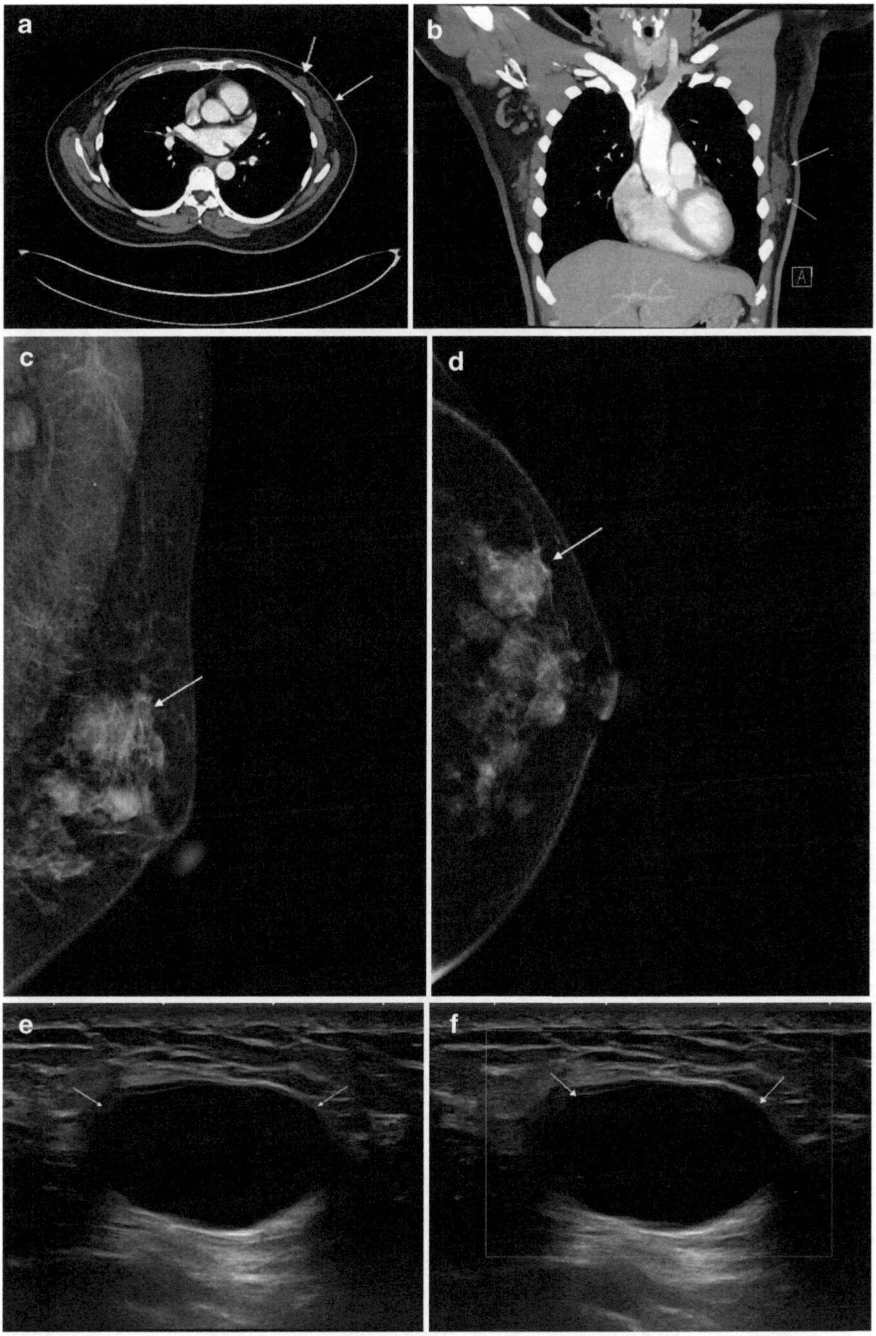

Fig. 2.6 Multiple breast cysts. Axial chest CT scan with IV contrast (**a**), coronal chest CT with IV contrast (**b**), mammography MLO view (**c**), CC view (**d**), grayscale ultrasound (**e**), and color Doppler (**f**) images. The chest CT image demonstrates several oval-circumscribed low-density masses in the left lateral breast (arrows). Multiple oval, circumscribed, isodense masses are observed on mammograms of the left breast, which correspond to typical anechoic benign cysts with posterior through transmission and no flow on color ultrasound. BI-RDAS 2 was given, and the patient was sent for routine age-appropriate screening

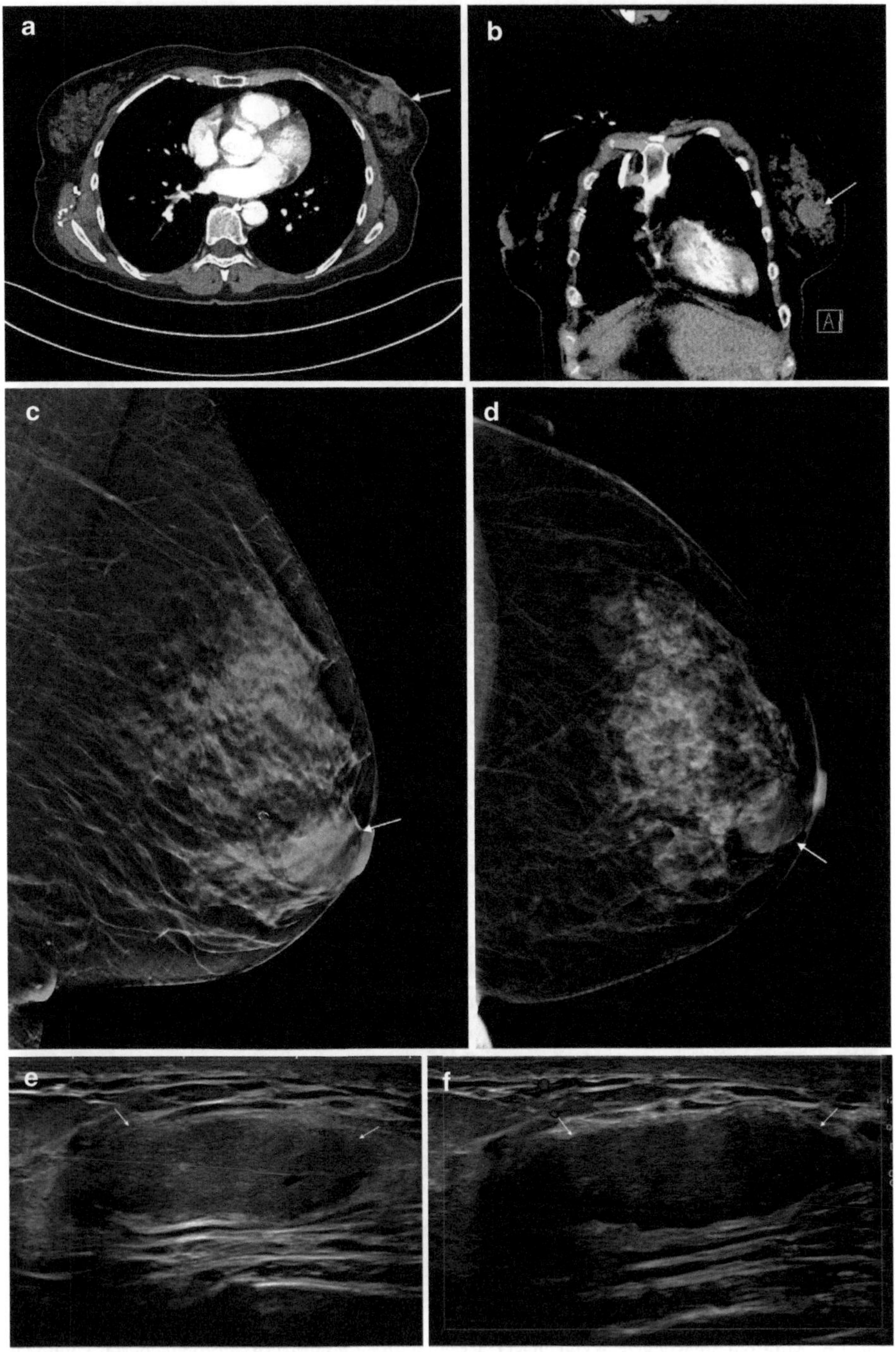
a
b
A
c
d
e
f

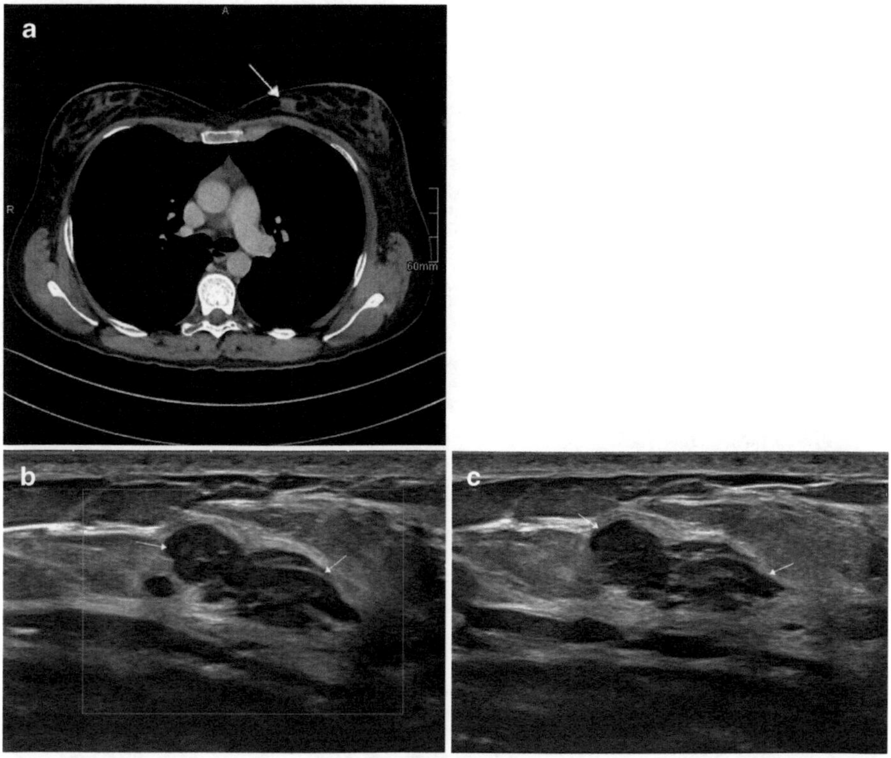

Fig. 2.8 Fibroadenoma with nonclassical imaging features. Axial CT chest with IV contrast (**a**), grayscale ultrasound (**b**), color Doppler ultrasound (**c**). Chest CT scan demonstrates a soft tissue mass with slightly irregular borders and mild enhancement in the left medial breast (arrow). Ultrasound confirmed a hypoechoic, hypovascular solid mass with some internal heterogeneity and microlobulated borders. Ultrasound-guided core biopsy was attempted and yielded a benign fibroepithelial lesion. Breast fibroadenomas are common benign breast tumours that are typically well-circumscribed; however, they may occasionally exhibit atypical features warranting further evaluation, including biopsy

Fig. 2.7 Pseudoangiomatous stromal hyperplasia (PASH). Axial CT chest with IV contrast (**a**), coronal reconstructed CT chest with IV contrast (**b**), mammography MLO view (**c**), CC view (**d**), grayscale ultrasound (**e**), and color Doppler ultrasound (**f**) of a patient with known colon cancer. Chest CT scan demonstrates an oval, circumscribed, slightly enhancing mass in the left retro nipple (arrow). Standard mammogram shows a partially circumscribed oval isodense mass with no associated suspicious calcifications (arrow). Ultrasound shows an oval, isoechoic, hypovascular solid mass with small internal cystic components. Ultrasound-guided core biopsy yielded benign breast tissue with dense stromal fibrosis and pseudoangiomatous stromal hyperplasia (PASH) with no evidence of atypia or malignancy, and a differential diagnosis of mass-forming PASH was suggested. While breast PASH is often a microscopic, incidental finding, it can also form a distinct mass. A precautionary short-term follow-up left breast imaging was recommended

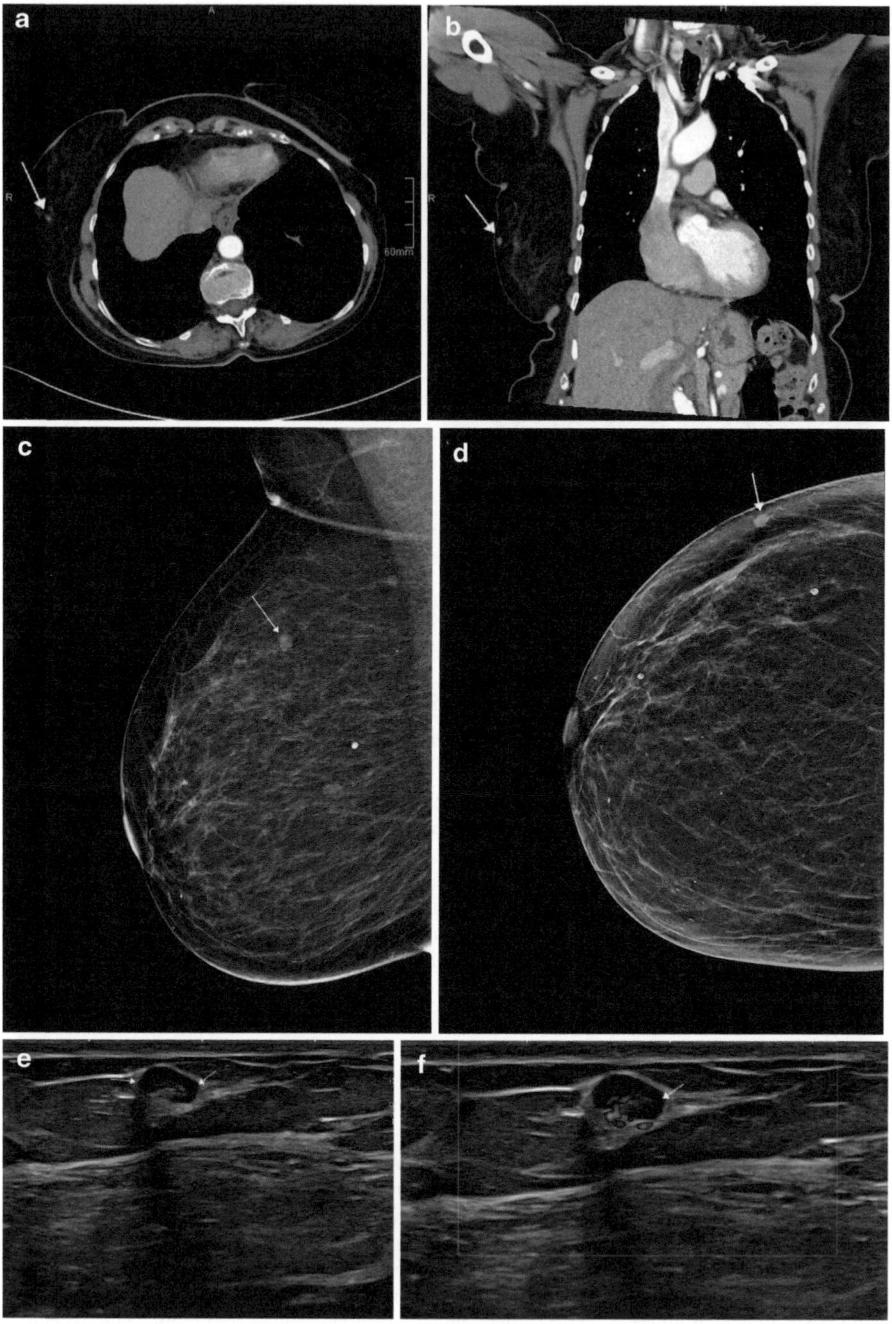

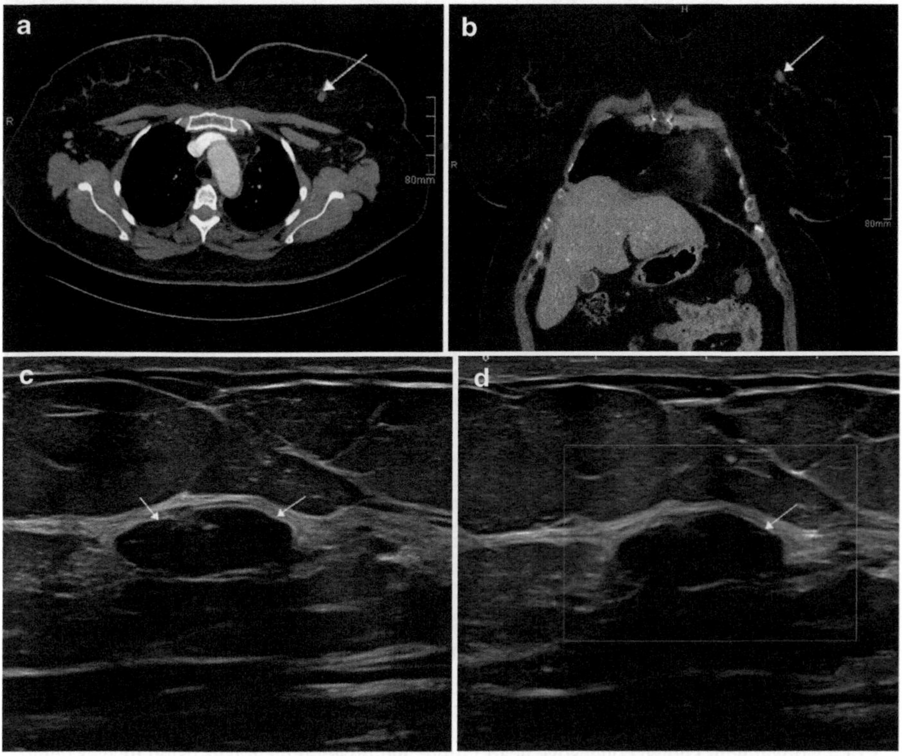

Fig. 2.10 Papilloma without atypia. Axial chest CT scan with IV contrast (**a**), coronal CT (**b**), grayscale ultrasound (**c**), and color Doppler ultrasound (**d**). Chest CT images demonstrate a circumscribed, oval, mildly enhancing soft tissue mass within the left upper central middle-posterior third breast (arrow). The mass appears homogeneous, hypoechoic, and hypovascular on the ultrasound (arrow). The mass was biopsied under ultrasound guidance and yielded a benign papilloma without atypia. The pathology was deemed concordant with radiology, and a short-term follow-up ultrasound was suggested, with no change in follow-up. Currently, in our centre, small (under 1 cm) radiologic–pathologic non-symptomatic concordant intraductal papillomas without atypia are managed with imaging follow-up rather than surgical excision

Fig. 2.9 Intermammary lymph node. Axial CT chest with IV contrast (**a**), coronal CT chest (**b**), mammography MLO view (**c**), CC view (**d**), grayscale ultrasound (**e**), and color Doppler ultrasound (**f**). Chest CT scan demonstrates an oval, small, circumscribed enhancing mass in the right upper outer breast (arrow). Two-view mammography demonstrated an oval, circumscribed, isodense mass in the upper outer posterior breast, which corresponded to a normal intermammary lymph node on ultrasound (arrow) (**e**). Color Doppler ultrasound showed the typical hilar flow of a lymph node. Routine age-appropriate screening mammography was suggested. An intramammary lymph node is a common benign breast finding that typically appears as a small, well-circumscribed oval or reniform mass with a preserved central fatty hilum, most often located in the upper outer quadrant

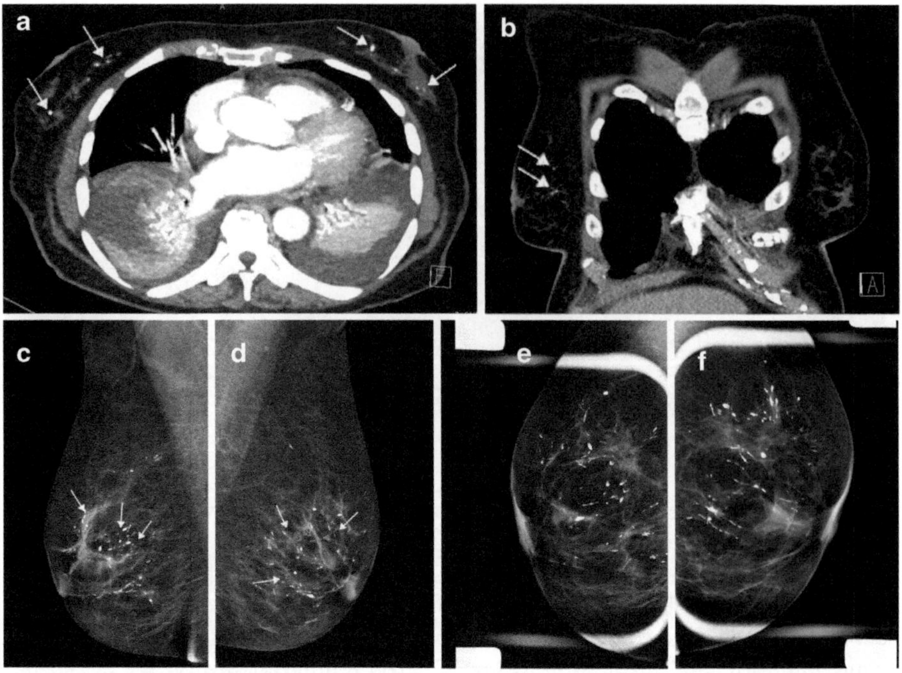

Fig. 2.11 Secretory calcifications. Axial chest CT scan MIP image with IV contrast (**a**), coronal CT (**b**), mammography MLO view right (**c**) and left (**d**), and focal compression views (**e**, **f**). Chest CT of a woman with known congestive heart failure and bilateral pleural effusion images demonstrate several round and rod-shaped calcifications scattered in the breasts (arrows). Mammography and additional focal magnification views show the same findings. Secretory-type calcifications due to plasma cell mastitis are mostly seen in post-menopausal women, and they are bilateral but usually asymmetric. The calcifications are generally larger than those of a malignant process. This is a benign entity; BI-RADS 2 can be assigned, and routine screening could be suggested

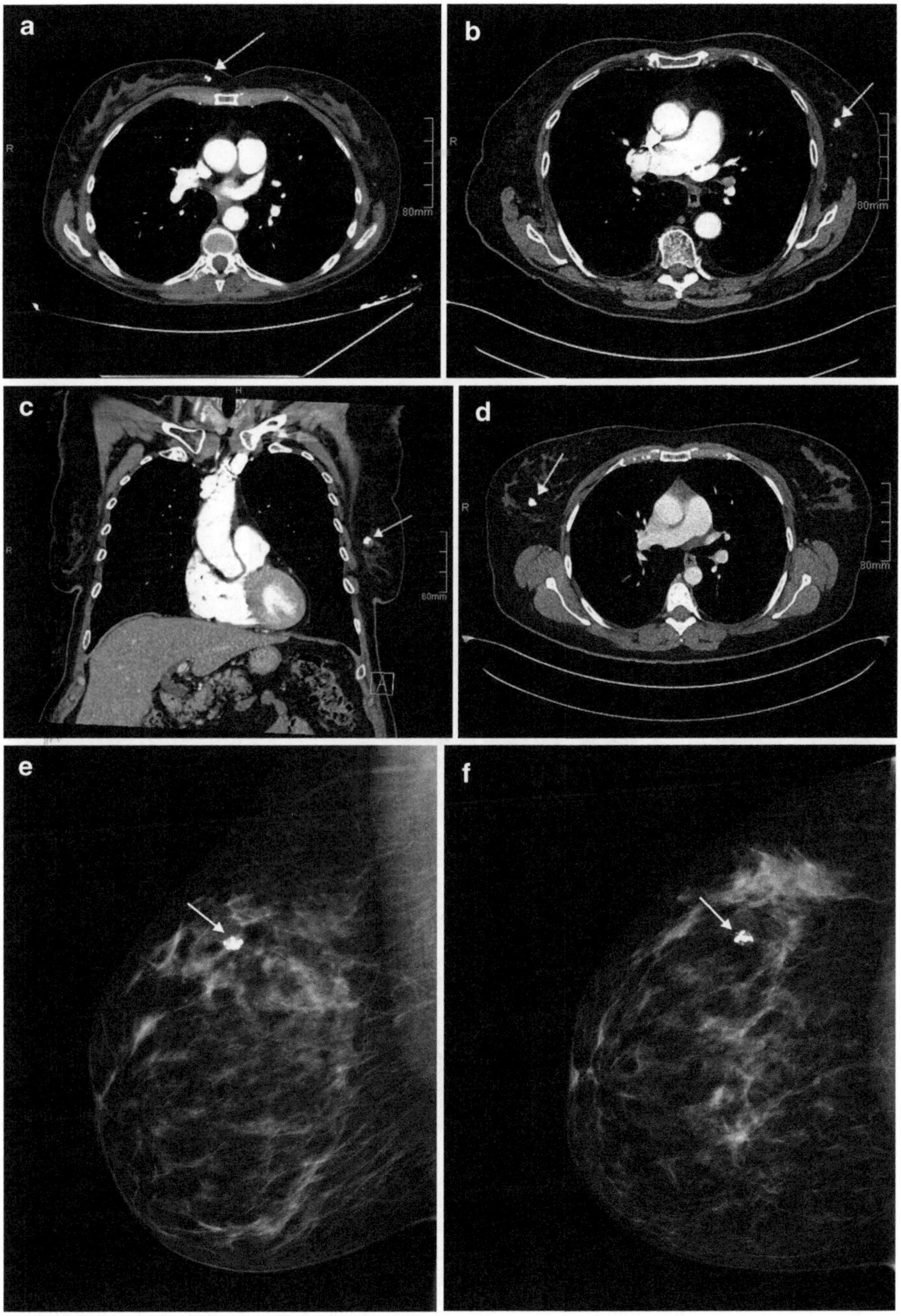

Fig. 2.12 Popcorn calcification. Axial chest CT scan with IV contrast (**a, b, d**) and a coronal chest CT scan (**c**) from different patients that reveal popcorn calcifications in the breasts (arrows). Images d to h belong to one case. Two-view right mammograms demonstrate a dystrophic calcification in the upper outer breast with an underlying mass (arrow). The findings correspond to an oval hypoechoic, nonvascular solid mass on ultrasound, with an internal bright echo. This type of calcification is indicative of degenerated fibroadenomas and is generally considered benign. BI-RADS 2 is given, and no further breast imaging follow-up is required

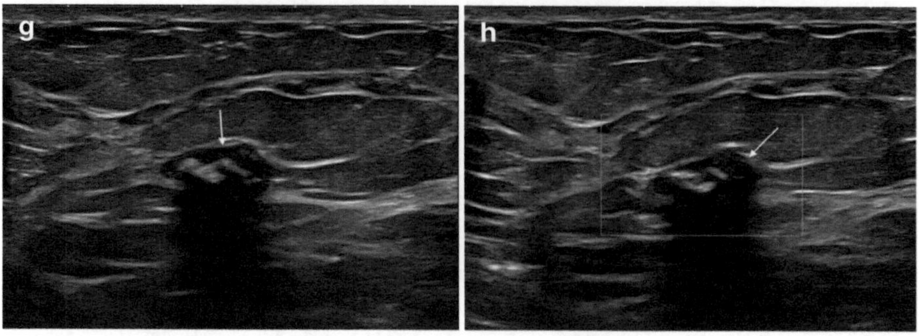

Fig. 2.12 (continued)

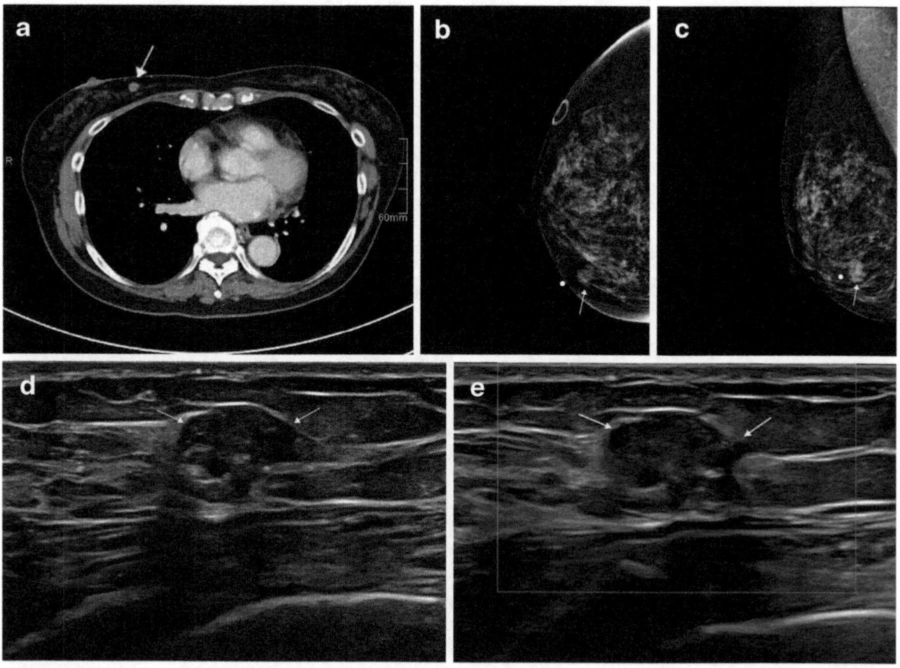

Fig. 2.13 Sclerosing papilloma. Axial chest CT scan with IV contrast (**a**), mammography CC view (**b**), MLO view (**c**), grayscale ultrasound (**d**), and color Doppler (**e**). Chest CT image demonstrates a circumscribed, oval, brightly enhancing mass within the right slightly lower inner breast (arrow) with a subtle central lucency. Mammography confirmed a partially obscured isodense mass in the same location, which was also palpable, and a BB marker was placed on the skin overlying the lesion. The ultrasound examination showed a lobulated, slightly heterogeneous, hypovascular, hypoechoic solid mass with internal cystic components. The mass underwent an ultrasound-guided core needle biopsy and yielded sclerosing papilloma with no atypia or malignancy. The patient opted for a surgical excision of the mass with no upgrade to malignancy results

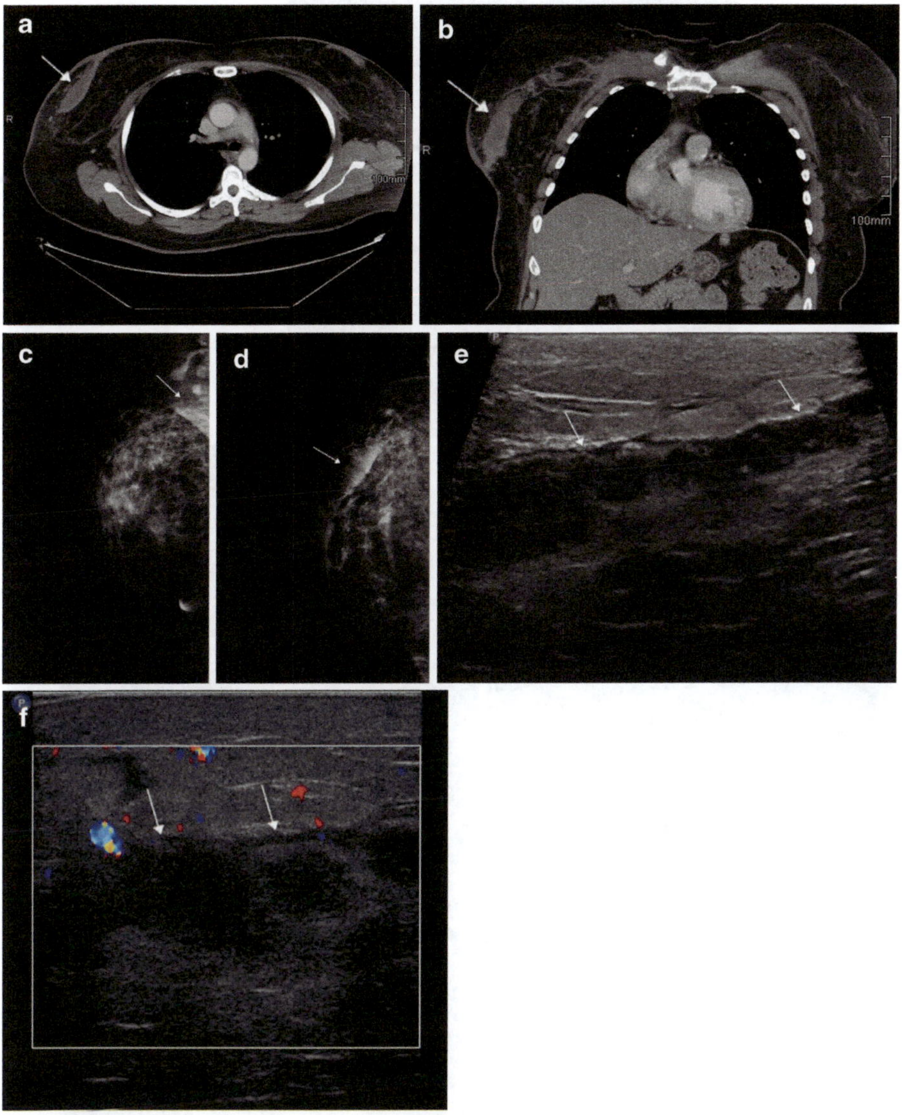

Fig. 2.14 Breast abscess. Chest CT scan with IV contrast axial and coronal (**a, b**), mammography MLO view (**c**), CC view (**d**), grayscale ultrasound (**e**), and color Doppler (**f**). Chest CT of a woman with a history of reduction mammoplasty reveals an elongated soft tissue mass with an internal fluid density and a peripheral rim enhancement located in the upper outer quadrant of the right breast (arrow). Mammography demonstrated a mass of similar shape and size at the same location, corresponding to the patient's swelling, skin redness, and induration. In the MLO view, there are some associated axillary tail prominent lymph nodes. Ultrasound examination revealed an oval mass containing fluid with debris, increased peripheral echogenicity, and hyperemia, suggestive of an abscess with surrounding inflammatory process. The patient underwent an ultrasound-guided fine-needle aspiration, during which pus was successfully aspirated. After aspiration of pus and antibiotic treatment, the abscess resolved, and the reactive axillary nodes became smaller

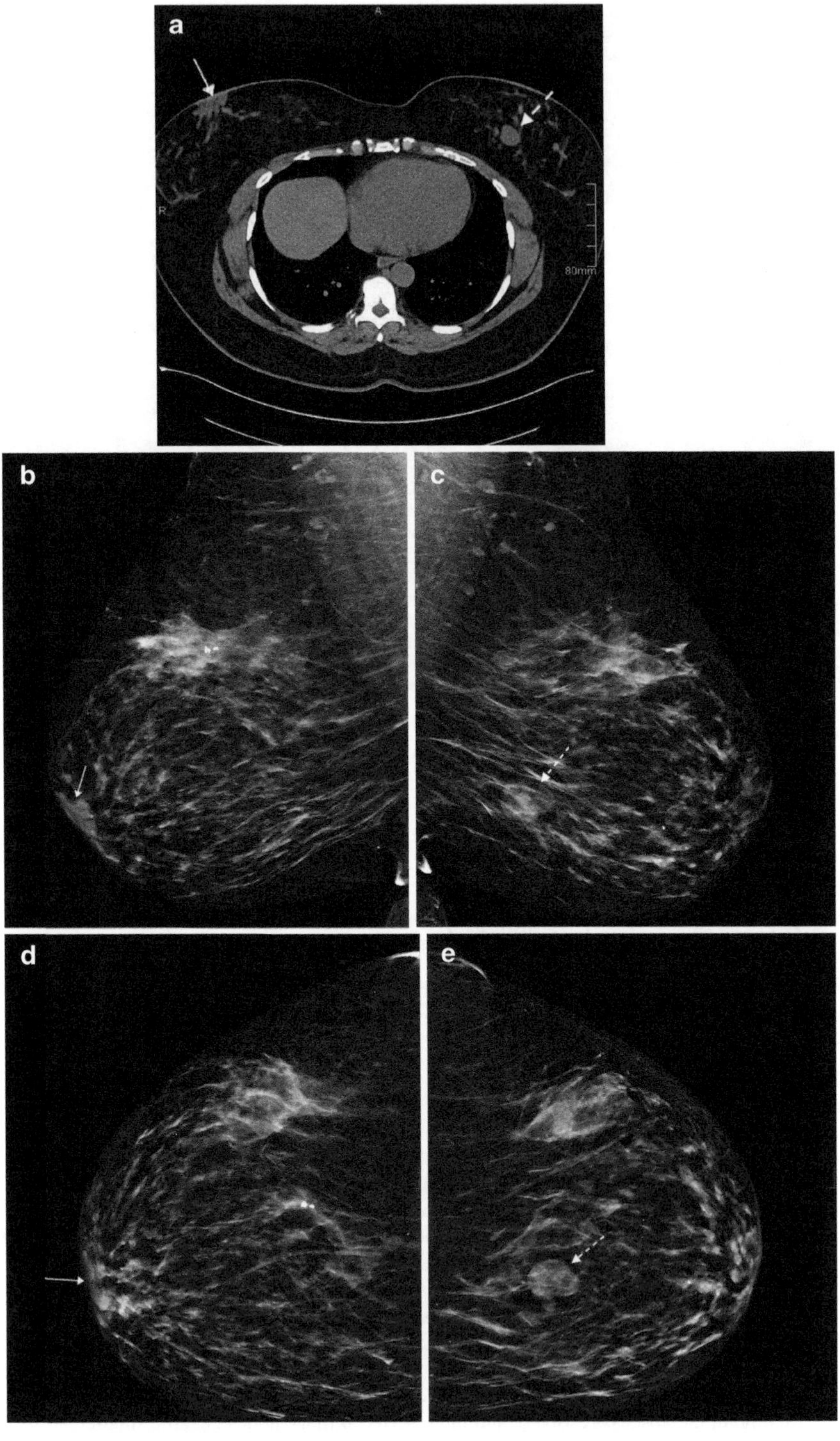

Fig. 2.15 Ductectasia and fibroadenoma. Chest CT scan without IV contrast axial (**a**), mammography MLO view right and left (**b, c**), CC view right and left (**d, e**), grayscale ultrasound (**f, g, h**),

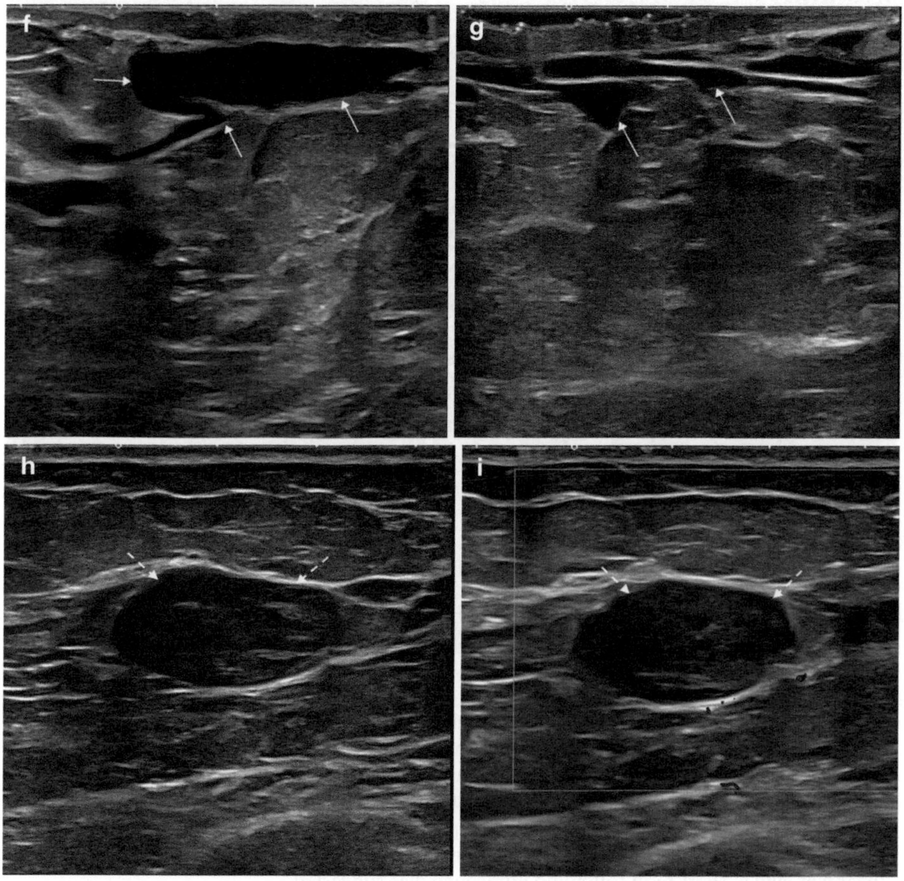

Fig. 2.15 (continued) and color Doppler (**i**). Chest CT reveals some tubular low-density structure behind the right nipple (solid arrow) and an oval, circumscribed soft tissue mass within the left breast, deep in the central breast (dashed arrow). Mammography with heterogeneous dense breasts demonstrated right retroareolar focal asymmetry, more tubular in CC view (solid arrow), and left central slightly lower deep breast circumscribed mass (dashed arrow). The ultrasound examination revealed right breast retroareolar duct ectasia with no intraductal solid mass and left circumscribed oval mass with mild internal heterogeneity, with low vascularity in color Doppler ultrasound. The mass had a remote benign biopsy, with a fibroadenoma result. A BI-RADS category 2 (benign findings) was assigned to the patient, and resuming routine screening was recommended

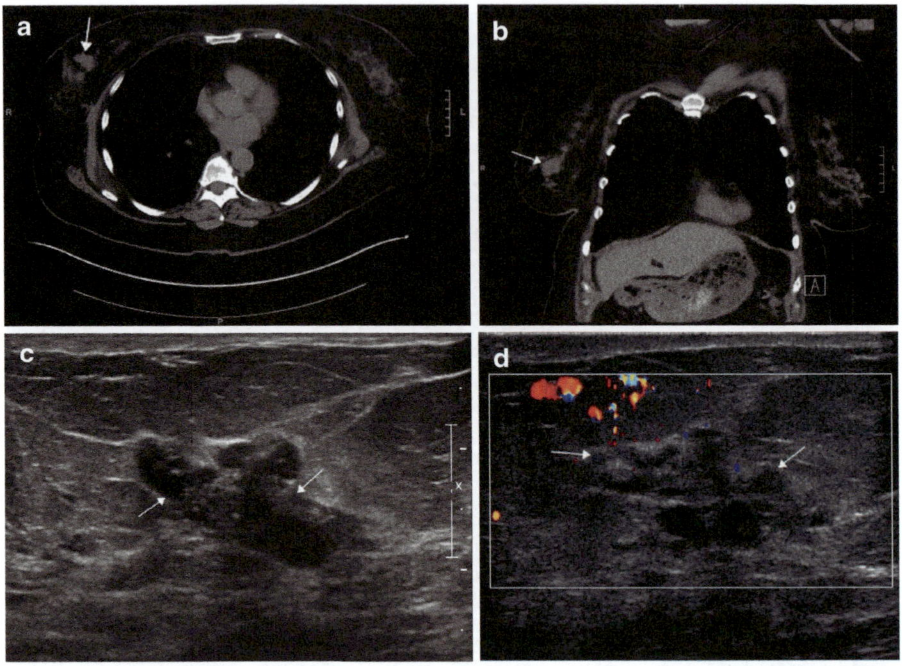

Fig. 2.16 Complex cyst. Chest CT scan with IV contrast axial (**a, b**), grayscale ultrasound (**c**), and color Doppler (**d**). Chest CT reveals a microlobulated soft tissue mass with subtle internal enhancing septa in the right central breast (solid arrow). The ultrasound examination revealed a right central breast complex cystic and solid mass with multiple internal cysts and thickened septa and low vascularity in color Doppler ultrasound. A BI-RADS category of 4 was assigned to the lesion. An ultrasound-guided core needle biopsy was performed, which revealed fibrocystic changes, columnar cell hyperplasia, and apocrine metaplasia. The pathology report was deemed concordant, and a short-term follow-up ultrasound was suggested

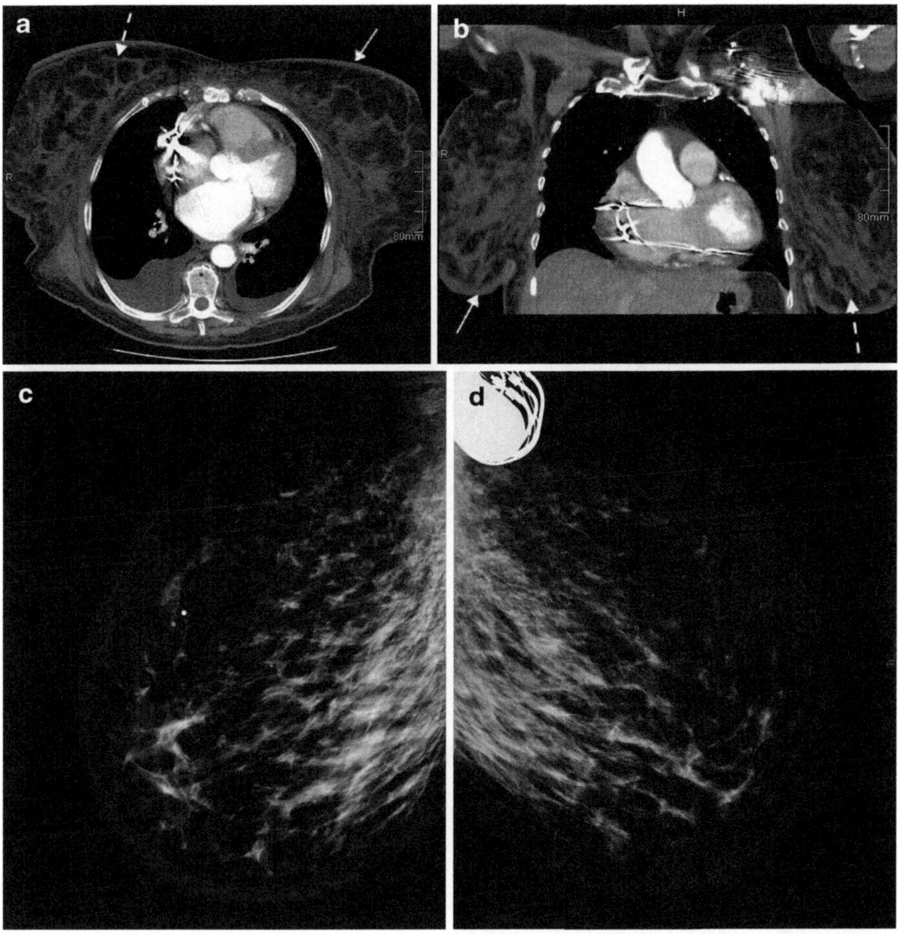

Fig. 2.17 Breast edema in congestive heart failure (CHF). Axial CT chest with IV contrast (**a**), coronal CT chest (**b**), mammography MLO view right and left (**c, d**), CC view right and left (**e, f**), and grayscale ultrasound (**g**). The chest CT revealed bilateral breast tissue edema, characterized by generalized swelling and enlargement, skin thickening (solid arrow), and increased thickening of Cooper's ligaments (dashed arrow). Additionally, a dual-lead pacemaker was noted in the left upper chest wall with its leads in the right heart chambers, along with bilateral pleural effusion. The patient has a documented history of heart failure. The ultrasound examination confirmed the CT findings, showing skin thickening (with measurement markers) and interstitial fluid consistent with edema. No further intervention regarding the breasts was deemed necessary, and routine screening was recommended. The patient remains under the care of cardiology

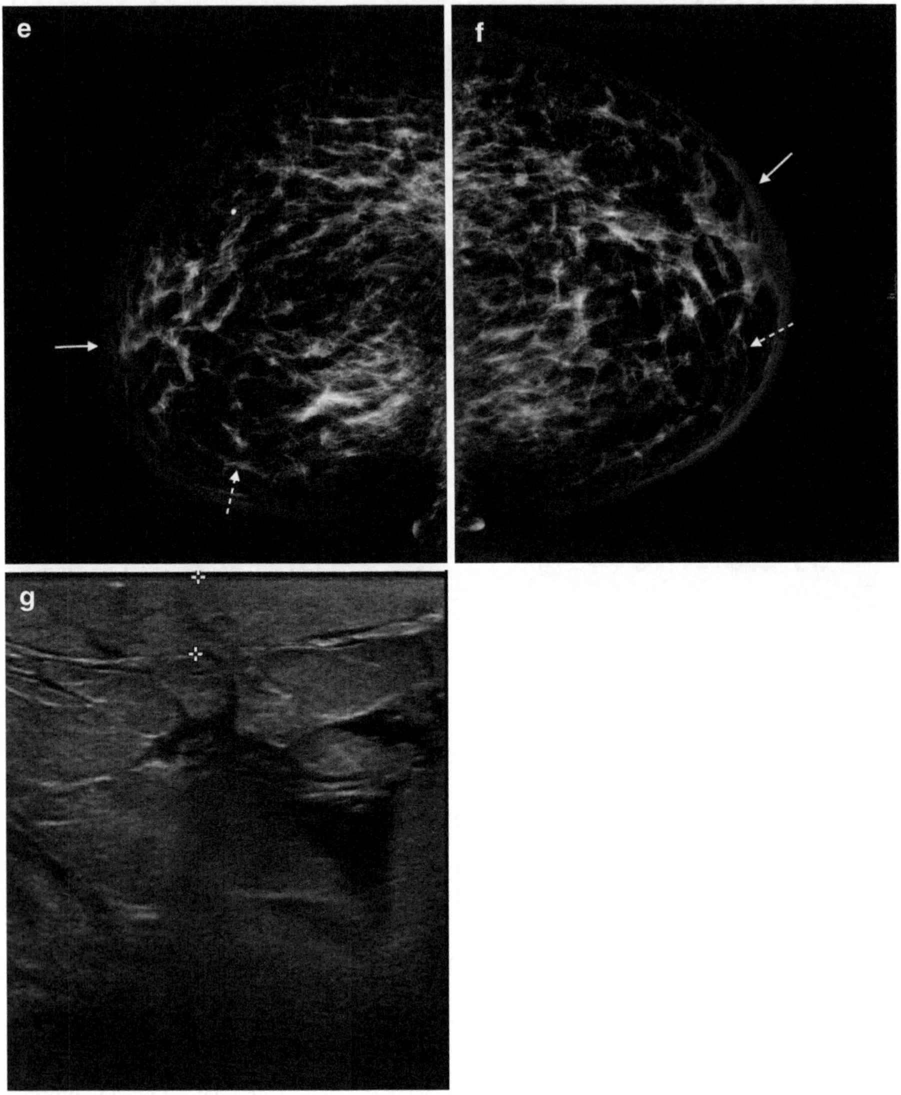

Fig. 2.17 (continued)

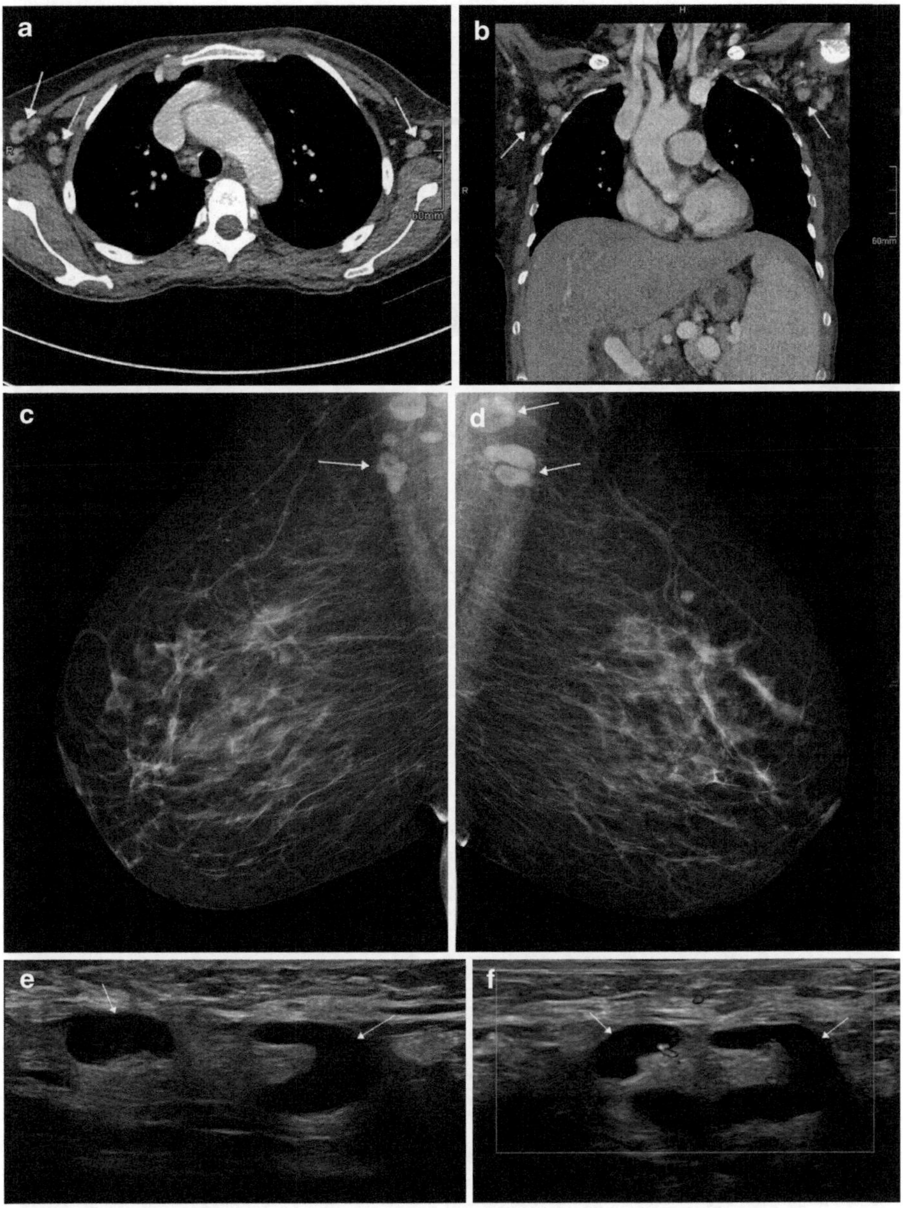

Fig. 2.18 Systemic lupus erythematosus (SLE). Axial CT chest with IV contrast (**a**), coronal CT chest (**b**), mammography MLO view (**c, d**), grayscale ultrasound (**e**), and color Doppler (**f**). The chest CT scan revealed prominent bilateral level 1 axillary lymph nodes (arrows), located lateral to the pectoralis minor muscles. Additionally, routine screening mammograms and MLO views showed enlarged axillary lymph nodes bilaterally (arrows). An ultrasound examination of the axillary regions confirmed the presence of large lymph nodes with preserved normal ultrasound morphology. These benign features include oval shape, an echogenic hilum, and normal hilar afferent and efferent vasculature, with no signs of neovascularization. These findings predominantly suggest that the lymph nodes are reactive. As a result, no further intervention regarding the breasts was deemed necessary, and routine screening was recommended. The patient has a history of systemic lupus erythematosus (SLE), which may explain the enlarged axillary nodes

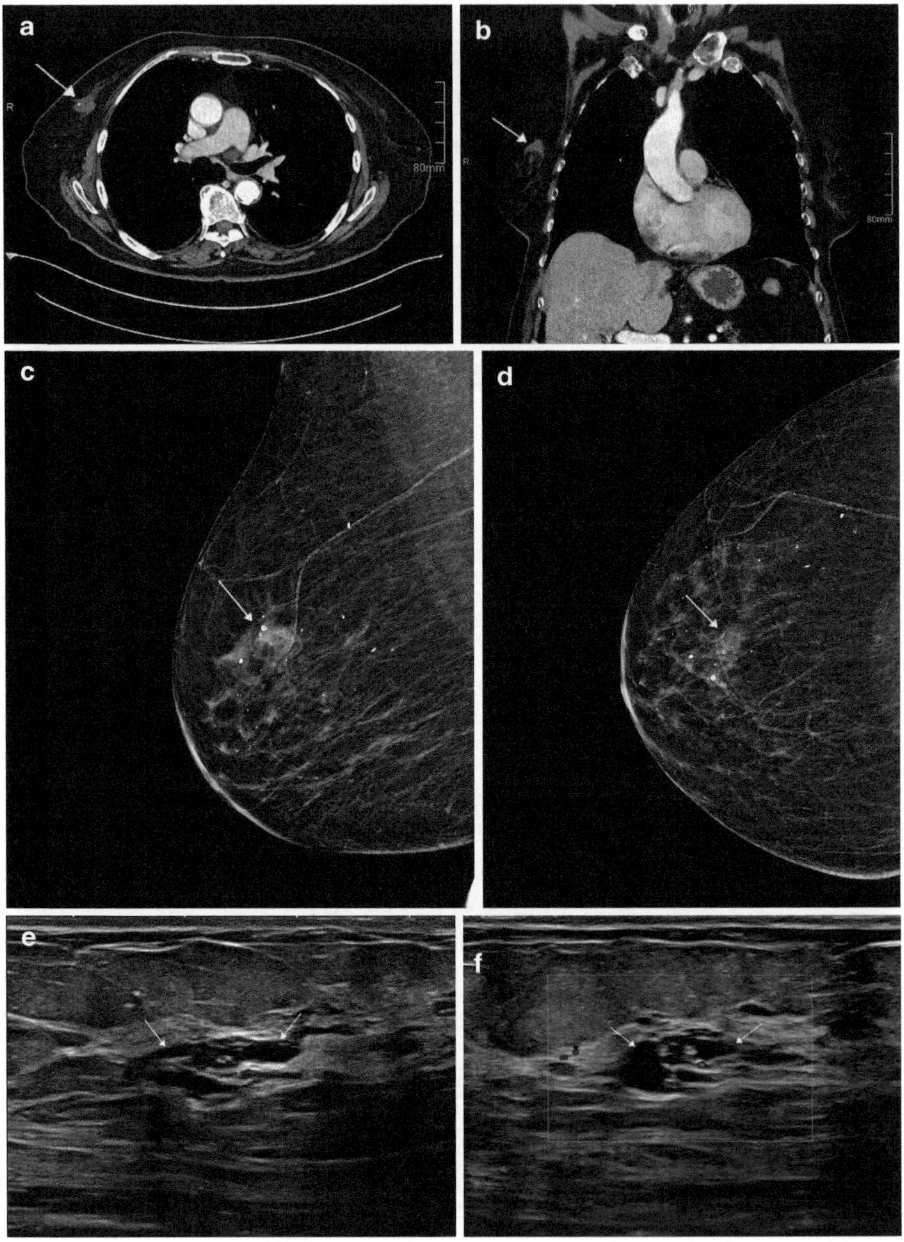

Fig. 2.19 Fibrocystic changes and atypical ductal hyperplasia. Axial CT chest with IV contrast (**a**), coronal CT chest (**b**), mammography MLO view (**c**), CC view (**d**), grayscale ultrasound (**e**), and color Doppler (**f**). The chest CT revealed a right upper slightly lateral breast irregular shape soft tissue mass with minimal enhancement and an associated round calcification (arrow). On two-view mammography, corresponding to the chest CT scan findings, there is a focal asymmetry in the right upper outer breast with several surrounding calcifications with benign morphology. The ultrasound examination showed clustered cysts without discrete solid components and minimal color flow on Doppler. An ultrasound-guided biopsy was conducted, which yielded fibrocystic changes and atypical ductal hyperplasia. Given the patient's age and comorbidities, she chose to pursue short--term follow-up instead of opting for excision of the lesion

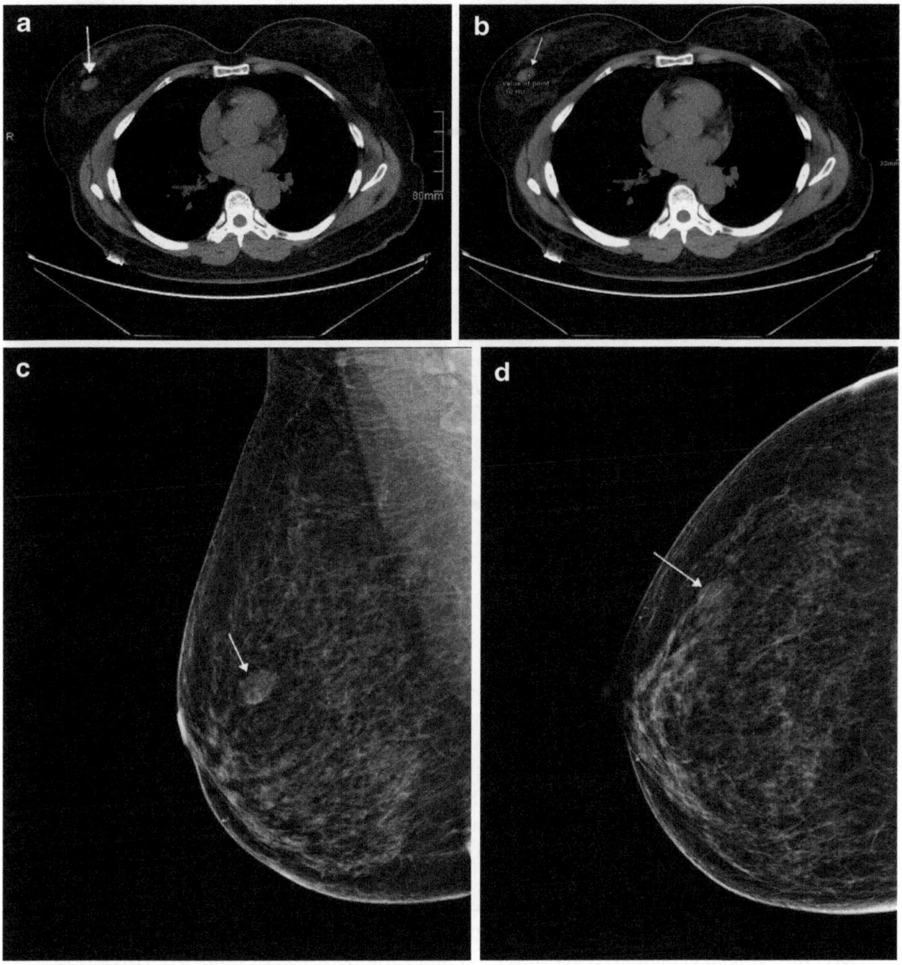

Fig. 2.20 Breast hamartoma or fibroadenolipoma. Axial CT chest without IV contrast (**a**, **b**), right breast mammography MLO view (**c**), CC view (**d**), focal compression spot view (**e**), grayscale ultrasound (**f**), and color Doppler ultrasound (**g**). The chest CT revealed a soft tissue oval mass in the right upper/slightly central, outer breast (solid arrow). There is a low-density area in the mass's medial portion, with a Hounsfield unit of −10, suggestive of macroscopic fat. Right breast mammography and compression spot views, corresponding to the chest CT scan findings, demonstrate an oval, low-density mass without calcifications or architectural distortion (arrow). The ultrasound examination confirmed an oval circumscribed mass with internal heterogeneous echogenic lines "Breast within Breast Appearance" (arrows) with no detectable flow in color Doppler evaluation. Overall, the findings are suggestive of a benign hamartoma or fibroadenolipoma. However, the patient opted for an ultrasound-guided core needle biopsy, which yielded the same results. The pathology results were considered concordant, and resuming routine screening mammography was recommended

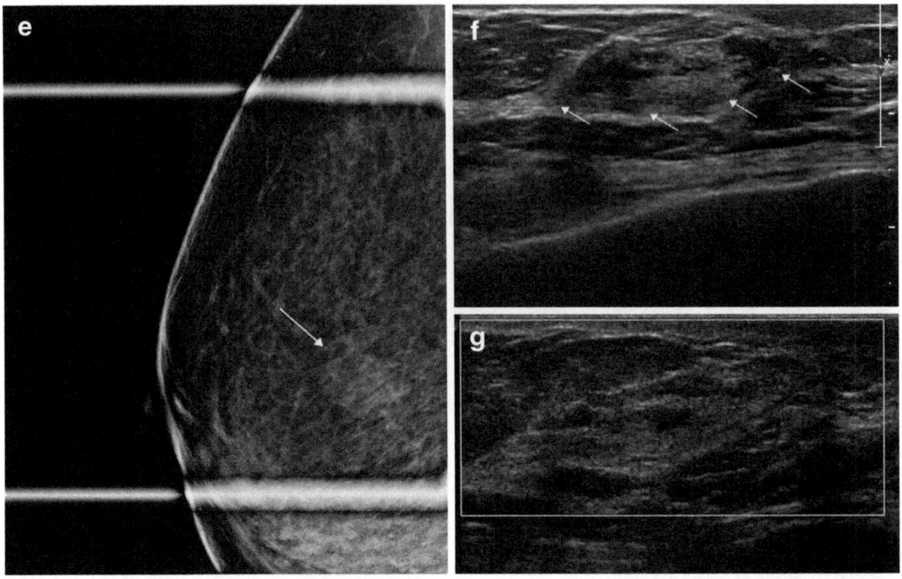

Fig. 2.20 (continued)

References

1. Choi YJ, Kim TH, Cha YJ, Son EJ, Gweon HM, Park CH. Incidental breast lesions on chest CT: clinical significance and differential features requiring referral. J Korean Soc Radiol. 2018;79(6):303–10. https://doi.org/10.3348/jksr.2018.79.6.303.
2. Harish MG, Konda SD, MacMahon H, Newstead GM. Breast lesions incidentally detected with CT: what the general radiologist needs to know. Radiographics. 2007;27(Suppl 1):S37–51. https://doi.org/10.1148/rg.27si075510.
3. Inoue M, Sano T, Watai R, Ashikaga R, Ueda K, Watatani M, Nishimura Y. Dynamic multidetector CT of breast tumors: diagnostic features and comparison with conventional techniques. AJR Am J Roentgenol. 2003;181(3):679–86. https://doi.org/10.2214/ajr.181.3.1810679.
4. Lam LY, Chu KM, Tsang HHC, Wai WC, Chiu JLF. The significance of computed tomography--detected breast lesions. Hong Kong J Radiol. 2024;27(3):e140–6. https://doi.org/10.12809/hkjr2317710.
5. Son JH, Jung HK, Song JW, Baek HJ, Doo KW, Kim W, et al. Incidentally detected breast lesions on chest CT with US correlation: a pictorial essay. Diagn Interv Radiol. 2016;22(6):514–8. https://doi.org/10.5152/dir.2016.15539. PMID: 27707680; PMCID: PMC5098945
6. Bin Saeedan M, Mobara M, Arafah MA, Mohammed TL. Breast lesions on chest computed tomography: pictorial review with mammography and ultrasound correlation. Curr Probl Diagn Radiol. 2015;44(2):144–54. https://doi.org/10.1067/j.cpradiol.2014.09.002.
7. Vachhani PG, Shah A, Fabrega-Foster K, Harvey S. Cysts with masses and masses with cysts: an imaging review of cystic breast masses. Appl Radiat Oncol. 2017;6(10):8–18.
8. Basara Akin I, Balci P. Fibroadenomas: a multidisciplinary review of the variants. Clin Imaging. 2021;71:83–100. https://doi.org/10.1016/j.clinimag.2020.11.036.

Chapter 3
Postoperative and Postinterventional Breast Changes on Chest CT

Understanding breast tissue changes after surgery (such as lumpectomy, mastectomy, or reconstruction) is crucial for radiologists to conduct effective follow-up imaging. Benign findings that are expected can sometimes resemble signs of recurrence; so recognizing these differences is key to minimizing false positives, unnecessary biopsies, and patient anxiety. Common postoperative imaging features include:

Skin Thickening and Edema These are frequently observed soon after surgery and generally resolve gradually over the following months.

Seroma This refers to a fluid collection in the surgical cavity, which can be identified as a well-defined area on ultrasound or as a fluid signal on MRI or CT scans.

Scar tissue: This appears as architectural distortion in the breast tissue.

Fat Necrosis Caused by disrupted blood supply to normal fatty tissue, fat necrosis can present in various forms, ranging from irregular masses to typical oil cysts.

Calcifications Dystrophic calcifications may develop over time at surgical sites, usually indicating benign changes.

Hematoma can present with variable morphology depending on its stage. Typically, it appears as a low-attenuation soft tissue mass in the breast, chest wall, or axilla. It has a higher attenuation in the early stages than serous fluid, but as it matures, it may resemble simple fluid. Notably, there should not be any enhancing solid soft tissue components. A reduction in the size of the hematoma over time is a reassuring sign [1–4].

These findings can change over time. Most acute changes, such as edema and seromas, are most noticeable within the first 6–12 months after surgery. In contrast, scar tissue and fat necrosis may persist or evolve beyond that timeframe [5–7].

A. Alikhassi, *Atlas of Breast Lesions on Chest Computed Tomography*,
https://doi.org/10.1007/978-3-032-22791-1_3

Breast imaging is typically performed using mammography, ultrasound, or MRI. However, chest CT scans are often conducted for unrelated reasons, such as trauma or respiratory symptoms, as well as for staging in oncology patients. To prevent misdiagnosis, it is crucial to understand the expected postoperative architecture and typical benign alterations when reading a postoperative breast on a CT scan.

Changes observed on chest CT scans in patients who have undergone breast surgery should be correlated with the patient's medical history and any prior breast imaging before deciding to recall the patient for further testing. Doing so can help mitigate unnecessary costs to the healthcare system and reduce anxiety for patients and their families [8].

Local or regional recurrence of breast cancer has been estimated to occur in 5–25% of patients who have undergone treatment. Local recurrence refers to the reappearance of a tumor at the surgical site. Chest CT scans, which provide cross-sectional images with high soft tissue resolution, are an excellent tool for evaluating breast cancer recurrence and potential involvement of the chest wall. Additionally, CT scans of the thorax can identify other important findings, such as pleural and pericardial effusions, as well as metastases in the bones, mediastinum, lungs, and liver, all of which are crucial for making treatment plans [9].

A thorough multimodal evaluation is required if any questionable results appear; this may involve a mammogram and targeted breast imaging for precise interpretation and treatment planning. Differentiating between postoperative alterations and actual pathology requires integrating the clinical timeline, surgical history, and evaluating prior breast imaging results.

Figures 3.1, 3.2, 3.3, 3.4, 3.5, 3.6, 3.7, 3.8, 3.9, 3.10, 3.11, 3.12, and 3.13 describe cases involving postsurgical interventional lesions.

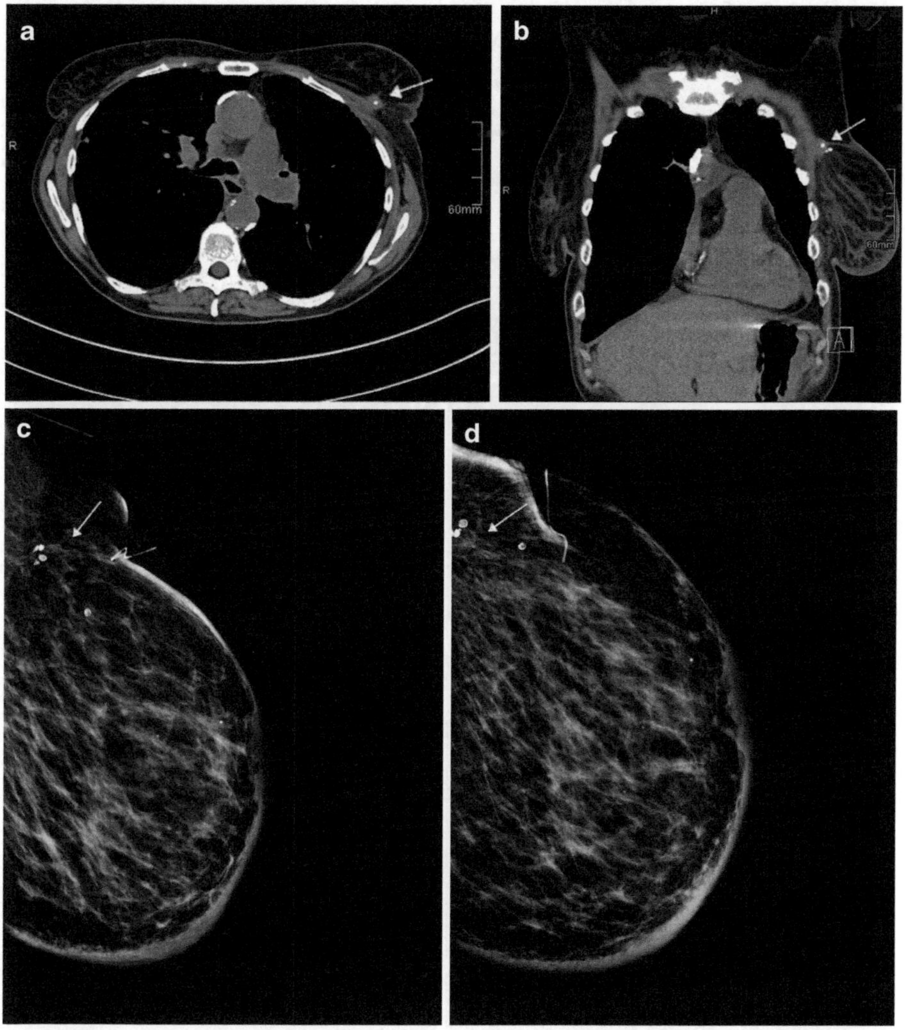

Fig. 3.1 Typical surgical breast scar. CT chest without IV contrast axial (**a**), coronal (**b**), mammography MLO view (**c**), and CC view (**d**) of a woman with a history of left breast lumpectomy and radiation. The chest CT scan showed signs of previous treatment, including thickening of the left breast skin and scar tissue in the upper outer breast region, along with a few round calcifications (arrow). The mammography findings showed typical scar tissue in the left breast and some round calcifications (arrow) in the posterior prepectoral region. A scar marker with dense linear metallic density was placed on the skin at the time of mammography to indicate the location of the scar. BI-RADS 2 was given, and a routine surveillance mammography was recommended

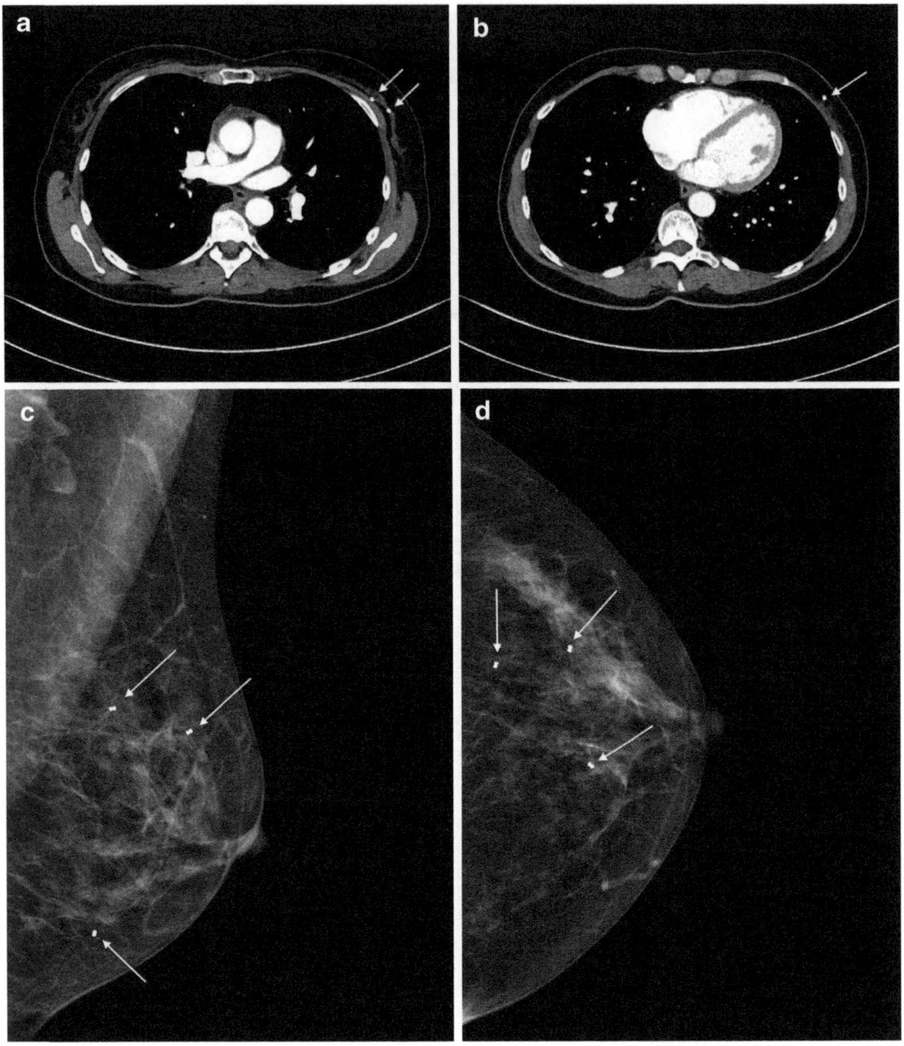

Fig. 3.2 Breast clips. Axial chest CT scan with IV contrast (**a, b**), mammography MLO view (**c**), and CC view (**d**). Chest CT demonstrates two metallic densities within the left lateral breast and one in the left slightly inner breast. Mammography revealed two marker clips in the upper outer quadrant of the left breast and one in the lower inner quadrant. The patient has a positive genetic test for the BRCA1 carrier mutation, placing her in the high-risk category. As part of the high-risk screening program, she had two annual MRI scans, which overall reported three suspicious findings. Following this, she had MRI-guided biopsies and clip placements, all of which resulted in benign pathologies. A breast marker clip is a small biocompatible marker placed at the biopsy site to permanently identify the area for future imaging follow-up or surgical localization

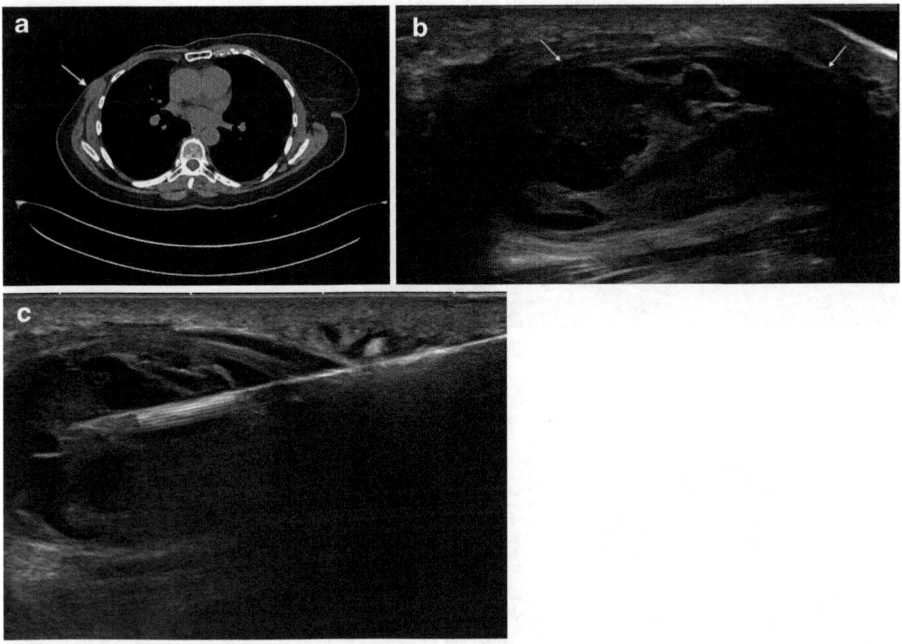

Fig. 3.3 Postmastectomy hematoma. Axial CT chest without IV contrast (**a**), grayscale ultrasound (**b**), and ultrasound-guided core biopsy (**c**). The chest CT scan of a woman with a recent right breast mastectomy revealed a soft tissue mass with a thick, denser rim and a lower-density center located in the right lateral chest wall. A right-sided chest wall ultrasound was also performed, which displayed a heterogeneous, cystic, non-vascular mass adjacent to the mastectomy scar, extending into the axillary tail. The differential diagnoses include an organized hematoma or seroma versus cancer recurrence. An ultrasound-guided biopsy was performed, and the results indicated benign scar tissue with mild chronic inflammation and fibrin, consistent with a hematoma

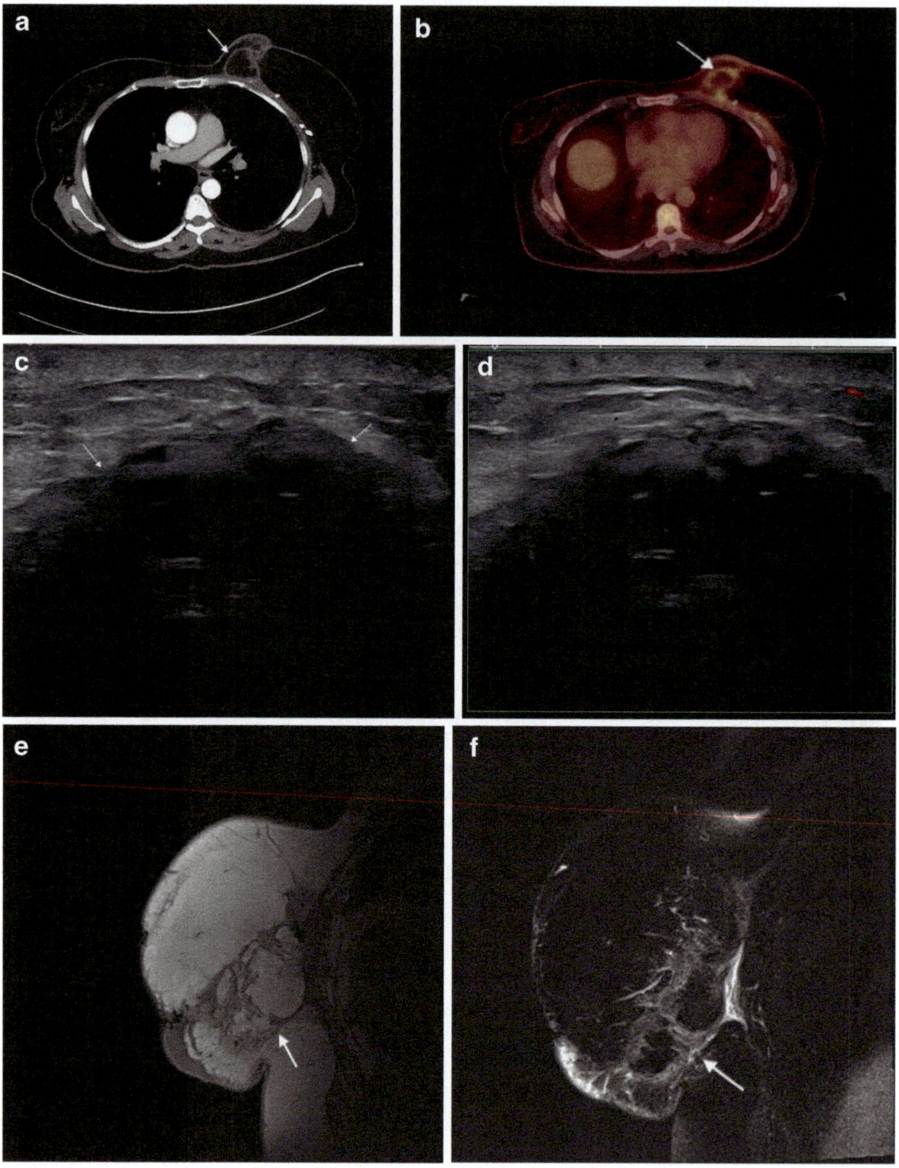

Fig. 3.4 Fat necrosis. Axial chest CT with IV contrast (**a**), PET scan (**b**), grayscale ultrasound (**c**), color Doppler ultrasound (**d**), sagittal T1-weighted non-fat-saturated non-contrast MRI (**e**), sagittal T2-weighted fat-saturated MRI (**f**), sagittal T1-weighted fat-saturated with contrast MRI (**g**), and axial T1-weighted fat-saturated with contrast MRI (**h**). The chest CT scan of a woman with a left breast mastectomy and DIEP flap reconstruction revealed a soft tissue mass with a thick, denser rim and central fat located in the left inner breast (arrow). PET scan showed mild peripheral radiotracer uptake. Ultrasound indicated a heterogeneous hypoechoic nonvascular mass in the same location. In MRI, the mass presented with central bright signal on T1-weighted images, which was suppressed in fat-saturated sequences, and it showed rim enhancement following contrast injection. The findings were reported typical for fat necrosis, and BI-RADS 2 was given

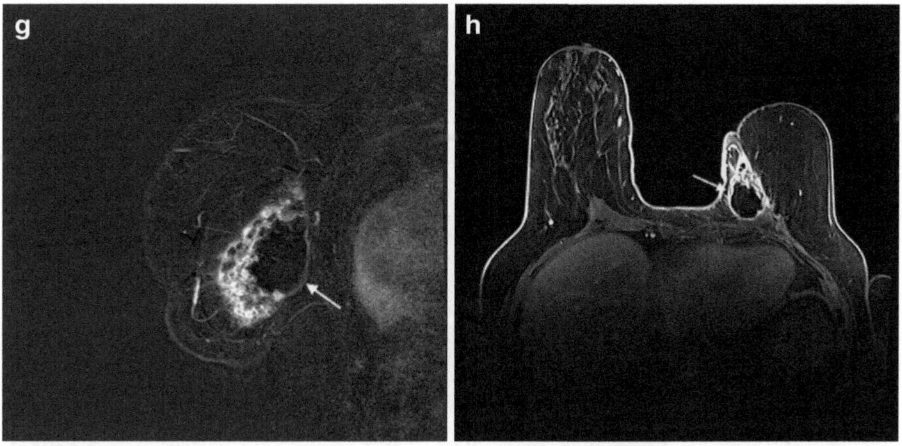

Fig. 3.4 (continued)

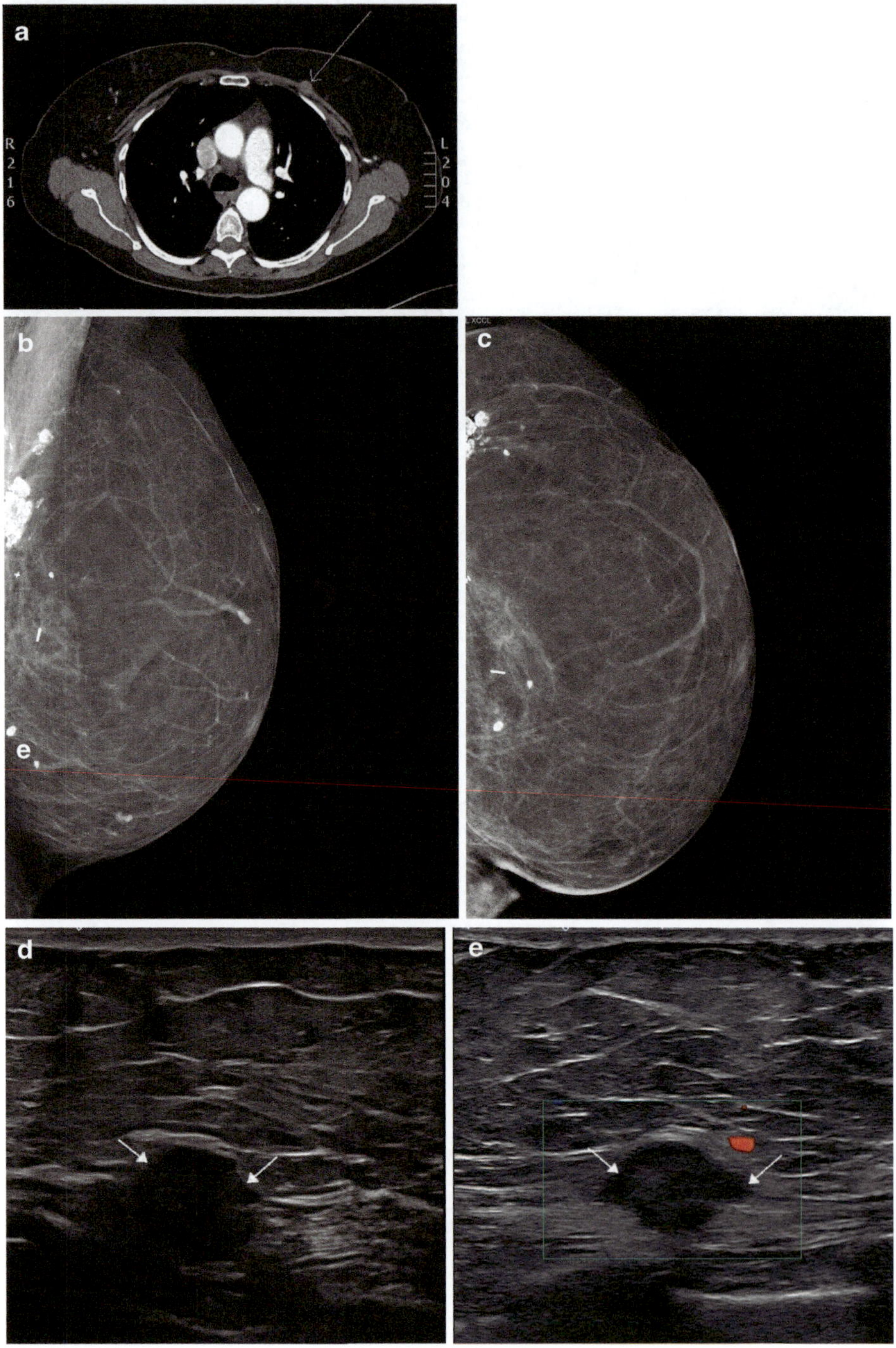
a
R
2
1
6
L
2
0
4
b
e
c
d
e

Fig. 3.5 Recurrence in TRAM flap reconstruction. Axial CT chest with IV contrast (**a**), mammography MLO view (**b**), CC view (**c**), ultrasound grayscale (**d**), and color Doppler ultrasound (**e**) of a woman with a history of left mastectomy, axillary dissection, radiation, and TRAM flap reconstruction. The chest CT scan revealed a deeply located, irregularly shaped peripherally enhancing mass in the mastectomy bed that involved the chest wall muscle (arrow). A subsequent mammogram showed that the left reconstructed breast is entirely composed of fatty tissue, with post-therapeutic changes related to the prior TRAM flap reconstruction. Additionally, benign dystrophic calcifications associated with fat necrosis were observed within the posterior left breast. However, the area of concern indicated on the CT chest, located within the left pectoralis muscle, was not visible on the mammogram due to its deep posterior position. Targeted ultrasound of the left reconstructed breast identified an irregular hypoechoic mass involving the chest wall muscle. The ultrasound-guided biopsy of the mass came as recurrent malignant ductal carcinoma

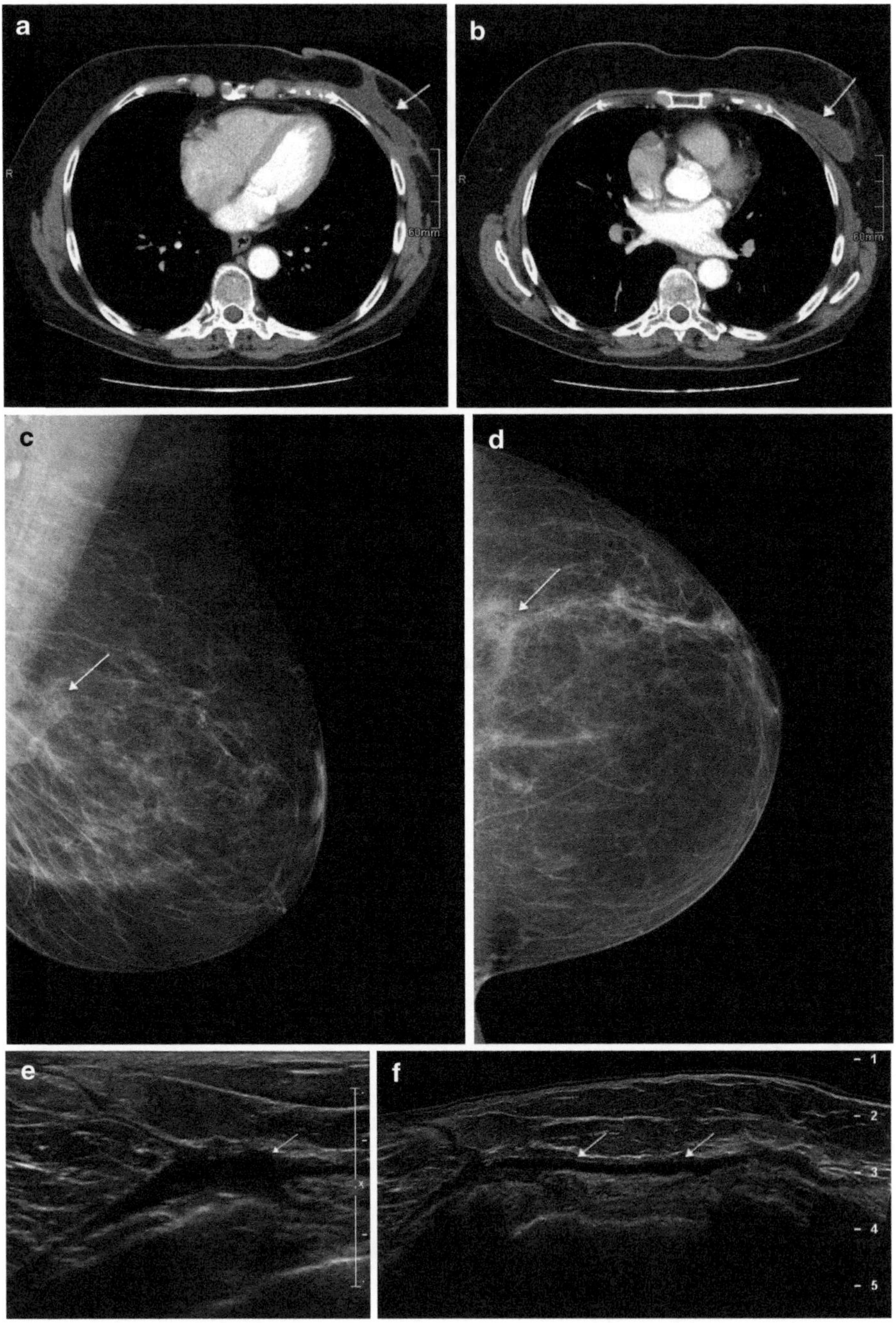

Fig. 3.6 Seroma. Axial CT chest with IV contrast (**a, b**), mammography MLO view (**c**), CC view (**d**), and grayscale ultrasound (**e, f**) of a woman with a history of recent left breast lumpectomy. Chest CT scan indicated a soft tissue low-density mass (HU < 20) in the left central posterior breast (arrow); the mass had a Hounsfield unit less than 20, consistent with fluid. The mammography findings showed scar tissue in the left breast associated with focal asymmetry in the posterior pectoral region. A targeted ultrasound of the area was performed and confirmed a surgical scar associated with fluid accumulation suggestive of seroma

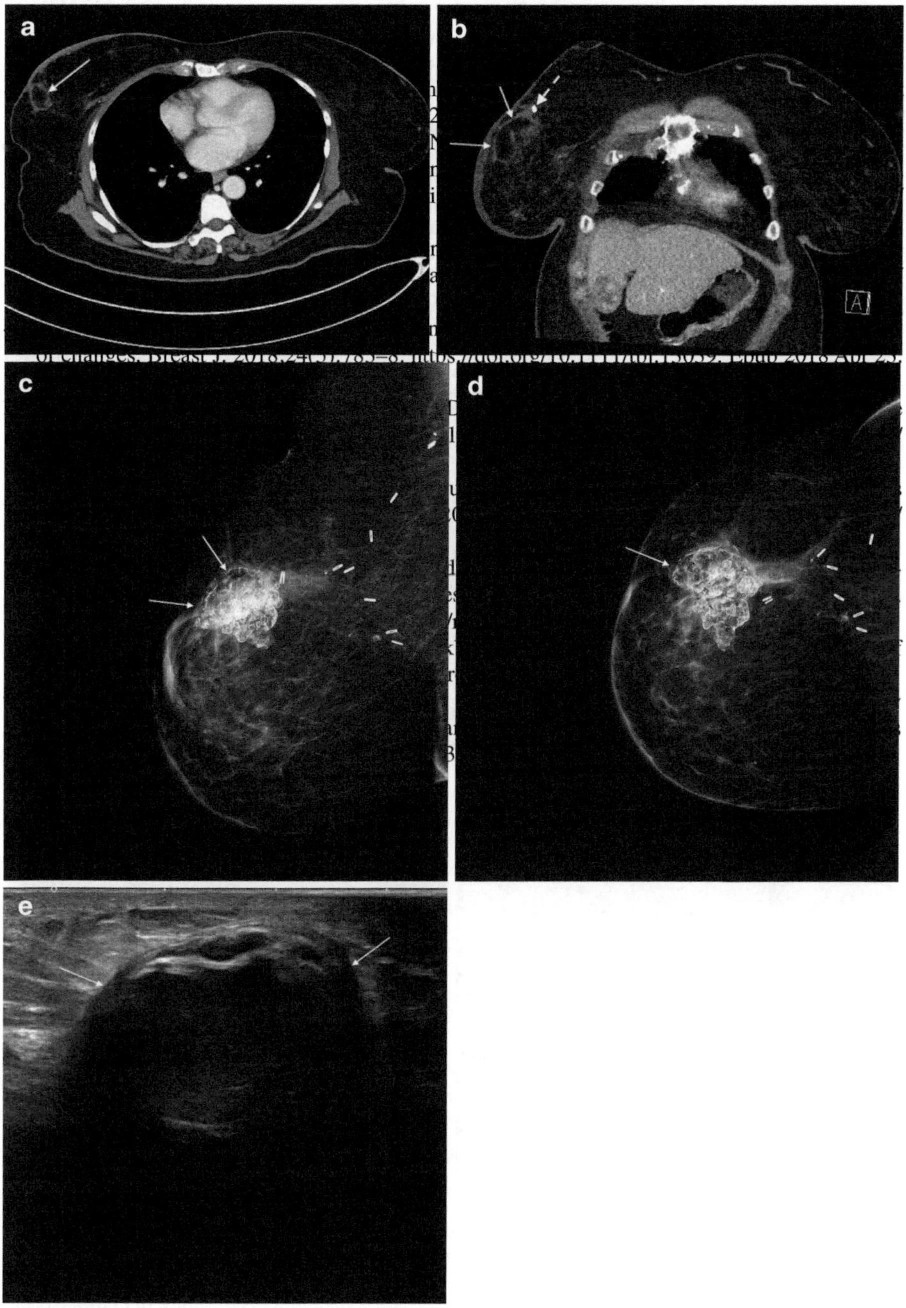

Fig. 3.7 (continued)

Fig. 3.7 Fat necrosis and oil cyst. Axial CT chest with IV contrast (**a**), coronal CT chest with IV contrast (**b**), mammography MLO view (**c**), CC view (**d**), and grayscale ultrasound (**e**) of a woman with a history of right lumpectomy and radiation. The chest CT scan revealed an oval, circumscribed mass with internal fat and a thin rim capsule containing calcifications (arrow); a surgical clip seen superior to the lesion in coronal image (dashed arrow). Mammogram showed postoperative changes, including scar and surgical clips in the upper outer quadrant, associated with a fat-containing mass with rim eggshell calcifications typical for fat necrosis (arrow). A targeted ultrasound identified an oval hypoechoic mass with an echogenic peripheral rim corresponding to the mammography calcifications. The findings were reported typical for fat necrosis and oil cysts; BI-RADS 2 was given, and a routine surveillance was suggested

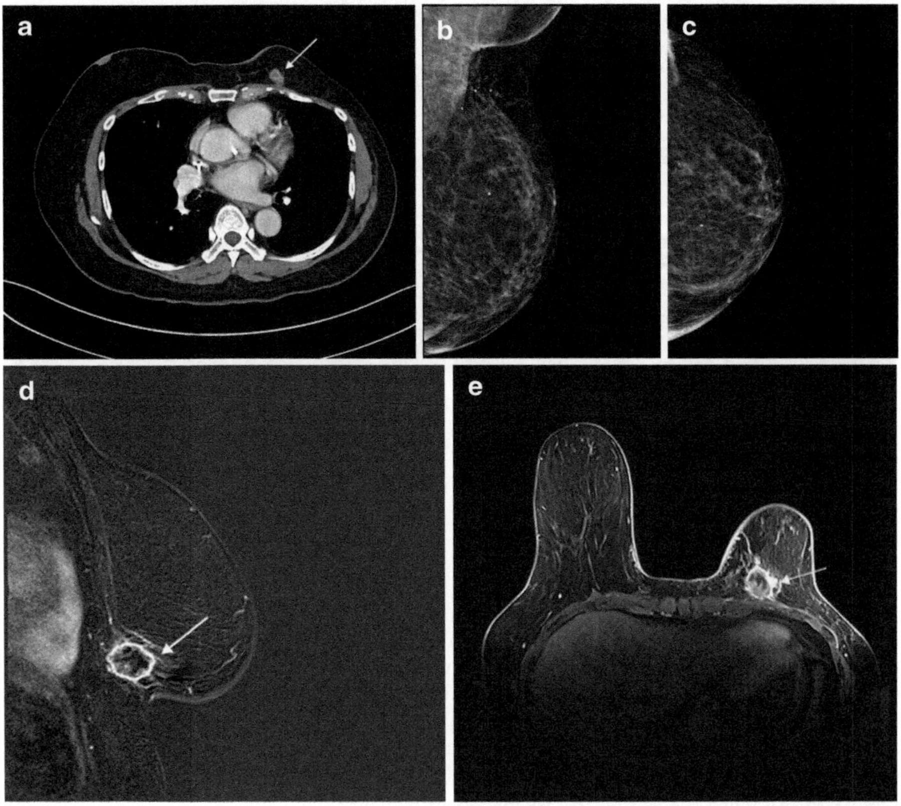

Fig. 3.8 Recurrence. Axial CT chest with IV contrast (**a**), mammography MLO view (**b**), CC view (**c**), sagittal fat-suppressed T1 weighted with contrast (**d**), and axial fat-suppressed T1 weighted with contrast images (**e**). Chest CT scan of a woman with a history of remote left breast lumpectomy and radiation demonstrates an irregular-shaped, rim-enhancing mass within the left posterior inner breast close to the chest wall. Standard left breast mammography does not show the mass, possibly due to posterior location. Breast MRI confirms the mass with rim heterogeneous enhancement, larger size, and chest wall involvement. Pathological analysis of the mass confirmed a recurrence of breast cancer

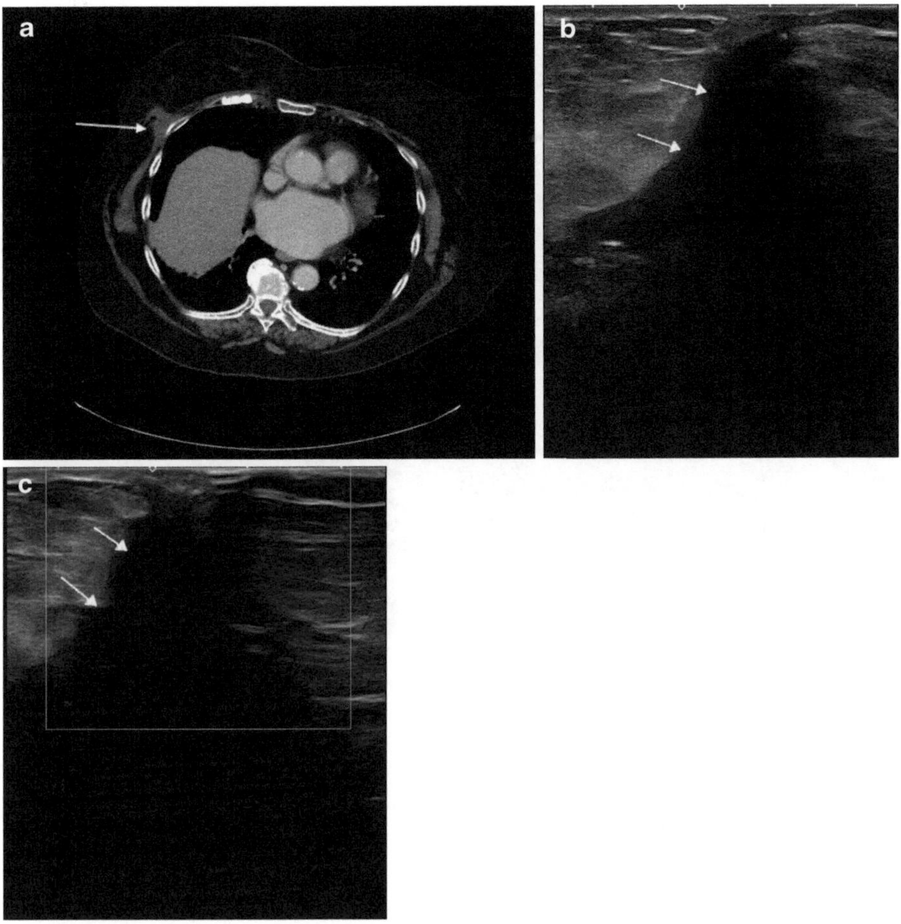

Fig. 3.9 Breast surgical scar. Axial CT chest with IV contrast (**a**), grayscale ultrasound (**b**), and color Doppler ultrasound (**c**) of a woman with a history of right breast lumpectomy, sentinel lymph node biopsy, and radiation therapy. Chest CT scan showed a triangular soft non/minimally enhancing soft tissue mass in the right lateral posterior chest area (arrow). Targeted ultrasound of the area was performed, and a non-mass hypoechoic nonvascular lesion extending to the skin was confirmed, suggestive of an unremarkable surgical scar. The patient was advised of routine surveillance. No change in the next surveillance was appreciated

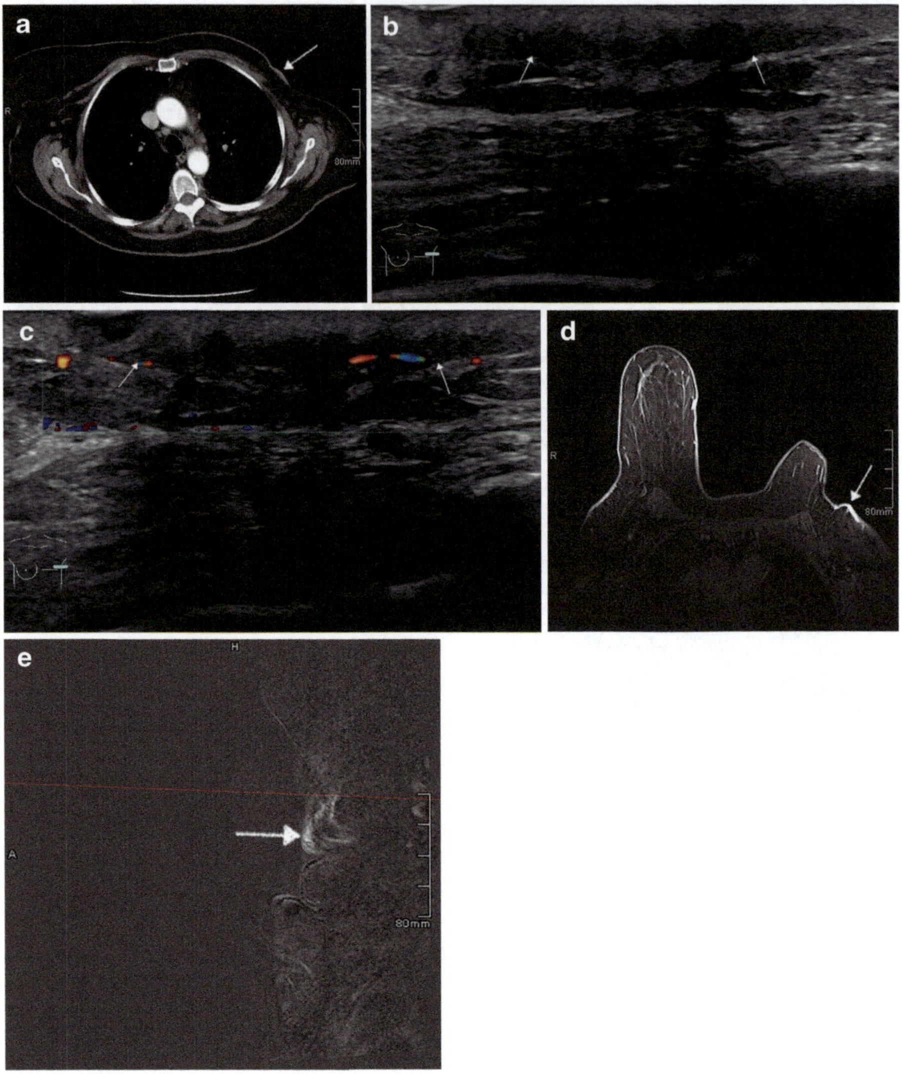

Fig. 3.10 Recurrence in skin. Axial CT chest with IV contrast (**a**), grayscale ultrasound (**b**), color Doppler ultrasound (**c**), and MRI T1 sequence with fat suppression and with IV contrast axial (**d**) and sagittal (**e**) of a woman with a history of remote left breast mastectomy. Chest CT scan indicated a new focal skin thickening of the left lateral chest wall (arrow). Ultrasound targeted to that area showed focal heterogeneous skin thickening with increased vascularity in color Doppler images. To further assess the posterior extent of the disease, an MRI was conducted, which also confirmed the pathologically enhanced focal skin thickening (arrow). A skin punch biopsy was performed, confirming a recurrence of breast cancer

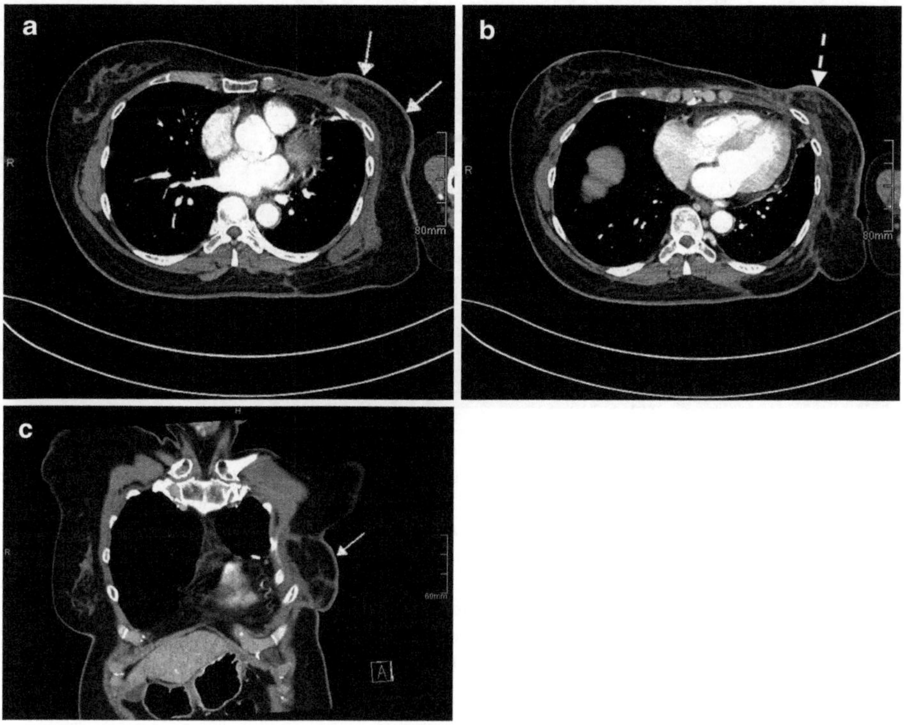

Fig. 3.11 Mastectomy and autologous flap reconstruction in chest CT scan. Axial CT chest with IV contrast (**a, b**), coronal (**c**) of a woman with a history of left breast mastectomy and flap reconstruction. The chest CT scan reveals that nearly all of the reconstructed breast is made up of fatty tissue, which differs from natural breast tissue and frequently has noticeable fatty streaks (arrow). Postoperative alterations (dashed arrow), surgical clips, and fat necrosis are typical concomitant findings. In flap reconstruction, the patient's own skin and subcutaneous fat are combined to create a pedicled or free tissue flap. In certain surgical methods, the breast mound may also be rebuilt using muscle from another part of the body

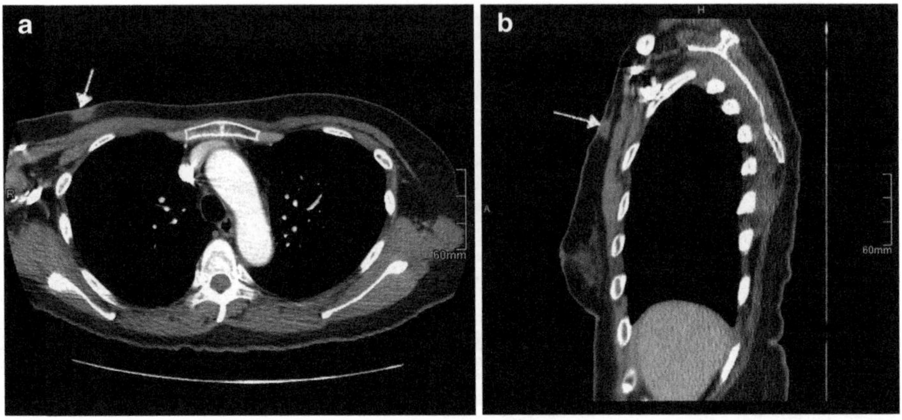

Fig. 3.12 Port-a-catheter hematoma. Axial CT chest with IV contrast (**a**), sagittal (**b**) of a woman with prior history of left breast cancer, lumpectomy, and radiation treatment. The chest CT scan revealed focal dermal and subdermal thickening in the right upper medial chest wall (arrow). Upon reviewing her medical history and the imaging results, it was noted that she had a port-a-catheter implanted in the right upper chest wall in the same location, as she had undergone chemotherapy. To reduce the chance of complications, a port-a-catheter is usually inserted beneath the skin in the upper chest on the side opposite the cancer, inferior to the clavicle. Chemotherapy, fluids, and blood draws are made simple by the catheter, which is inserted into the superior vena cava vein close to the heart, eliminating the need for frequent arm needle punctures

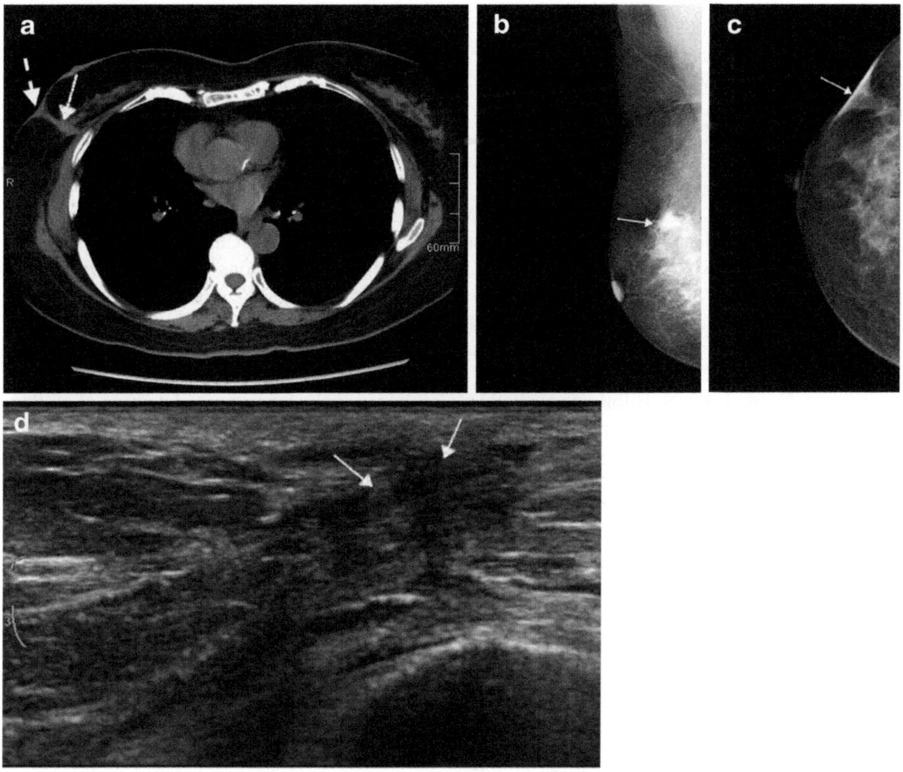

Fig. 3.13 Breast lumpectomy scar. CT chest without IV contrast axial (**a**), mammography MLO view (**b**), CC view (**c**), and grayscale ultrasound (**d**) of a woman with a history of right breast lumpectomy and radiation. The chest CT scan showed a linear soft tissue density (arrow), extending from the prepectoral region to the skin (dashed arrow), typical of a surgical scar. The mammography findings showed typical scar tissue in the right upper outer breast (arrow) without any discrete mass or calcifications. BI-RADS 2 was given, and a routine surveillance mammography was recommended

Chapter 4
Male Breast Findings on Chest CT

Breast pathology is significantly more prevalent in women, but male breast diseases are an important yet often overlooked clinical and radiological challenge. With the increased number of chest CT scan requests and greater access to imaging technology, radiologists are increasingly facing a larger spectrum of male breast diseases. It is vital to understand the typical imaging findings of these disorders for proper diagnosis and timely treatment. The normal adult male breast typically consists of a small, rudimentary amount of breast tissue, consisting primarily of adipose tissue (fat), atrophic ducts, and stromal elements located in the subareolar region, making abnormalities easier to detect when present [1, 2].

The typical male breast lacks the lobular units found in female breasts and is mostly made up of subcutaneous fat and primitive ductal systems. As men do not have lobules, they usually do not get lobular-based disorders such as lobular cancer, fibroadenomas, or lobular hyperplasia. However, ductal proliferation can be stimulated by hormonal imbalances, specific drugs, hereditary abnormalities, and systemic disorders, resulting in both benign and malignant diseases [3].

Male breast disorders encompass a broad spectrum of benign and malignant conditions, each with unique imaging features. The majority of cases are gynecomastia, but malignancy, while rare, should always be addressed, particularly in older men or when imaging findings raise suspicion. Mammography and ultrasound are vital for evaluation, helping to guide subsequent intervention and care. Although male breast cancer accounts for less than 1% of all breast cancer occurrences, delayed detection is prevalent due to poor clinical suspicion and the absence of screening programs. Early detection of specific imaging abnormalities is critical to prevent misdiagnosis and ensure prompt treatment [4].

In contrast to gynecomastia, malignancy is more likely to show as a unilateral, eccentric, non-retroareolar tumor with irregular or spiculated borders. Associated findings of malignancy may include nipple retraction, microcalcifications (which are less common compared to women), and skin thickening. On ultrasonography,

A. Alikhassi, *Atlas of Breast Lesions on Chest Computed Tomography*,
https://doi.org/10.1007/978-3-032-22791-1_4

malignant tumors often appear hypoechoic and irregular, often with angular or spiculated margins and posterior acoustic shadowing [5–7].

Gynecomastia appears on CT as a flame-shaped or nodular retroareolar density that enhances similarly to soft tissue. Malignancy, in contrast, may present as a discrete, irregular, or spiculated mass eccentric to the nipple, sometimes accompanied by skin thickening, nipple retraction, or axillary lymphadenopathy. CT is particularly useful in evaluating the local extent of advanced disease, detecting chest wall invasion, or identifying distant metastases. Because many CT-based breast findings are incidental, radiologists must maintain vigilance, recommending targeted mammography or ultrasound for further characterization when suspicious features are present [8, 9].

Figures 4.1, 4.2, 4.3, 4.4, 4.5, 4.6, 4.7, 4.8, 4.9, 4.10, 4.11, 4.12, 4.13, and 4.14 present a comprehensive collection of male breast lesions, encompassing a spectrum from benign to malignant conditions. Each series of figure describes a case illustrated with dedicated mammography and sonography images and along with final pathology results if needed, allowing readers to follow the diagnostic pathway from chest CT to final diagnosis. This case-based structure serves as a practical resource for understanding imaging patterns and establishing differential diagnoses in male breast diseases.

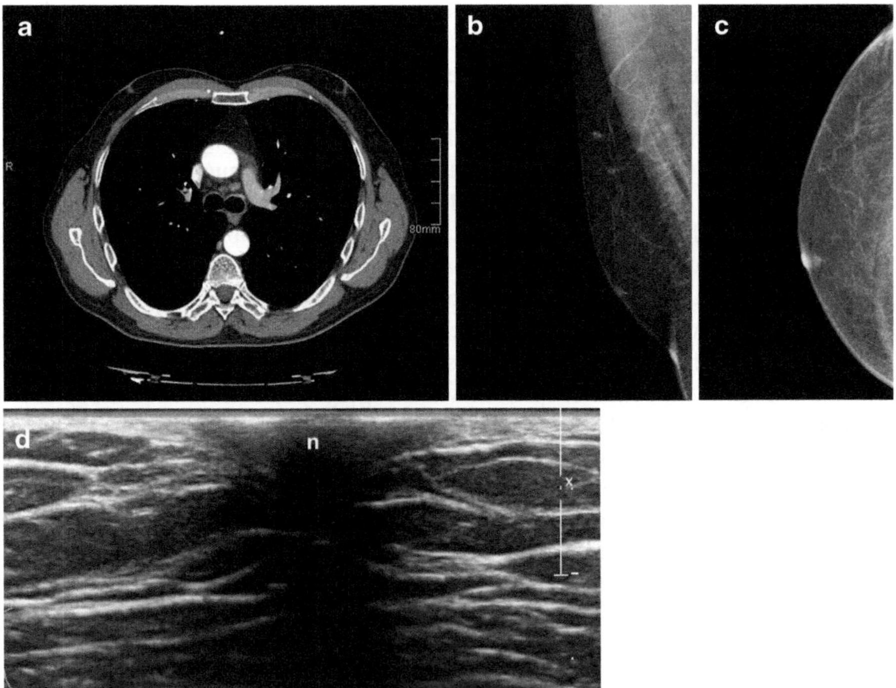

Fig. 4.1 Normal male breast. Axial chest CT scan with IV contrast (**a**), mammography MLO view (**b**), CC view (**c**), and ultrasound grayscale (**d**). Normal male breasts in different modalities are shown. N in the image (**d**) demonstrates the nipple

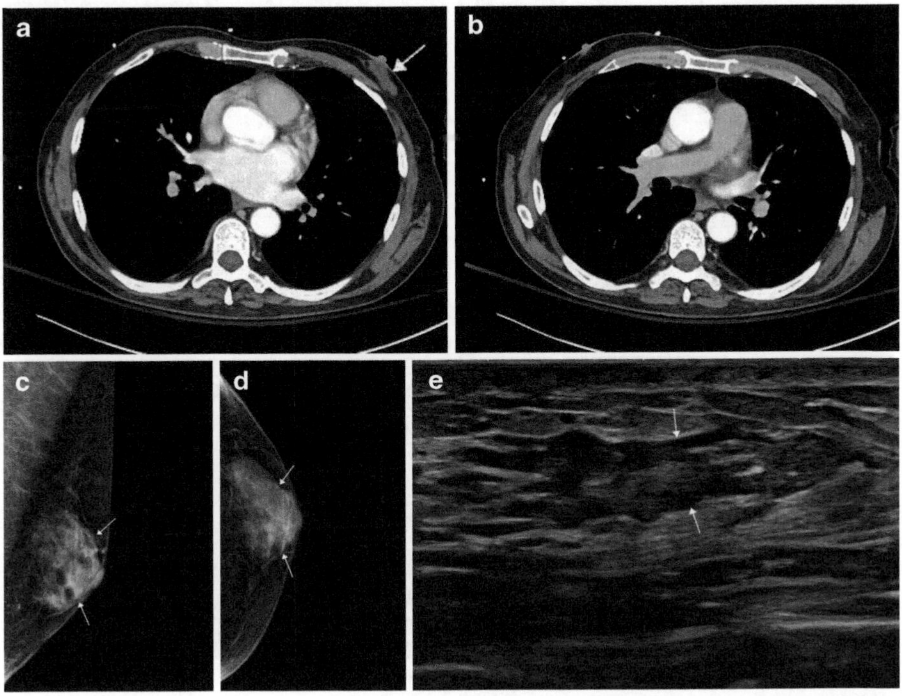

Fig. 4.2 Gynecomastia. Axial chest CT scan with IV contrast (**a, b**), mammography MLO view (**c**), CC view (**d**), and grayscale ultrasound (**e**). The chest CT scan (**a**) revealed asymmetrical non-mass soft tissue within the left central breast (arrow) and normal male breast on the right side (**b**). The mammogram showed increased fibroglandular tissue in the left central retroareolar breast. In the ultrasound, a flame-shaped, non-mass hypoechoic lesion located in the central retro nipple, typical for gynecomastia, corresponds to the chest CT scan and mammography findings

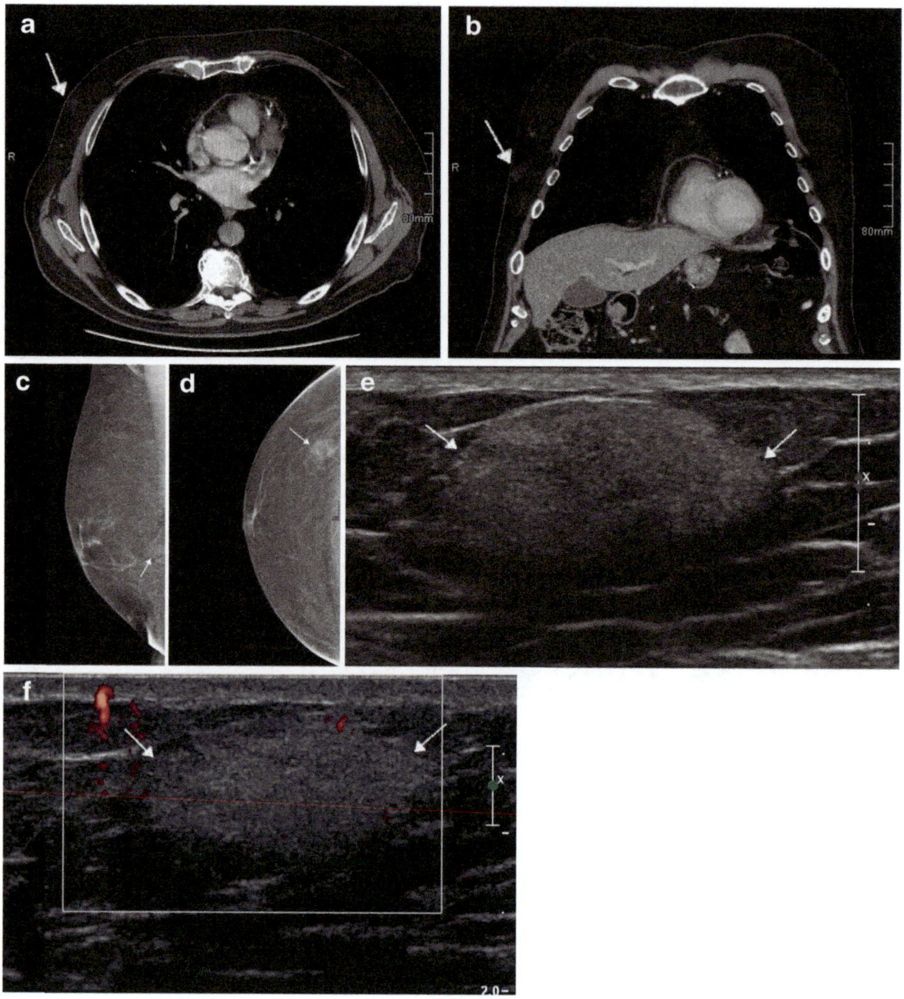

Fig. 4.3 Angiolipoma of male breast. Axial CT chest without IV contrast (**a**), coronal view (**b**), right breast mammography MLO view (**c**), CC view (**d**), grayscale ultrasound (**e**), and color Doppler ultrasound (**f**). The chest CT in a male patient revealed a faint soft tissue oval mass in the right lower lateral subdermal breast (arrow). The mass has some low-density internal components with a Hounsfield unit of less than −10, suggestive of macroscopic fat. Right breast mammography, corresponding to the chest CT scan findings, demonstrates an oval mass with mixed fat and soft tissue densities and without calcifications or architectural distortion (arrow). The ultrasound examination confirmed a superficially located oval, circumscribed, echogenic mass with mild vascularity on color Doppler. The mass underwent an ultrasound-guided biopsy and yielded angiolipoma, a benign, rare male breast pathology

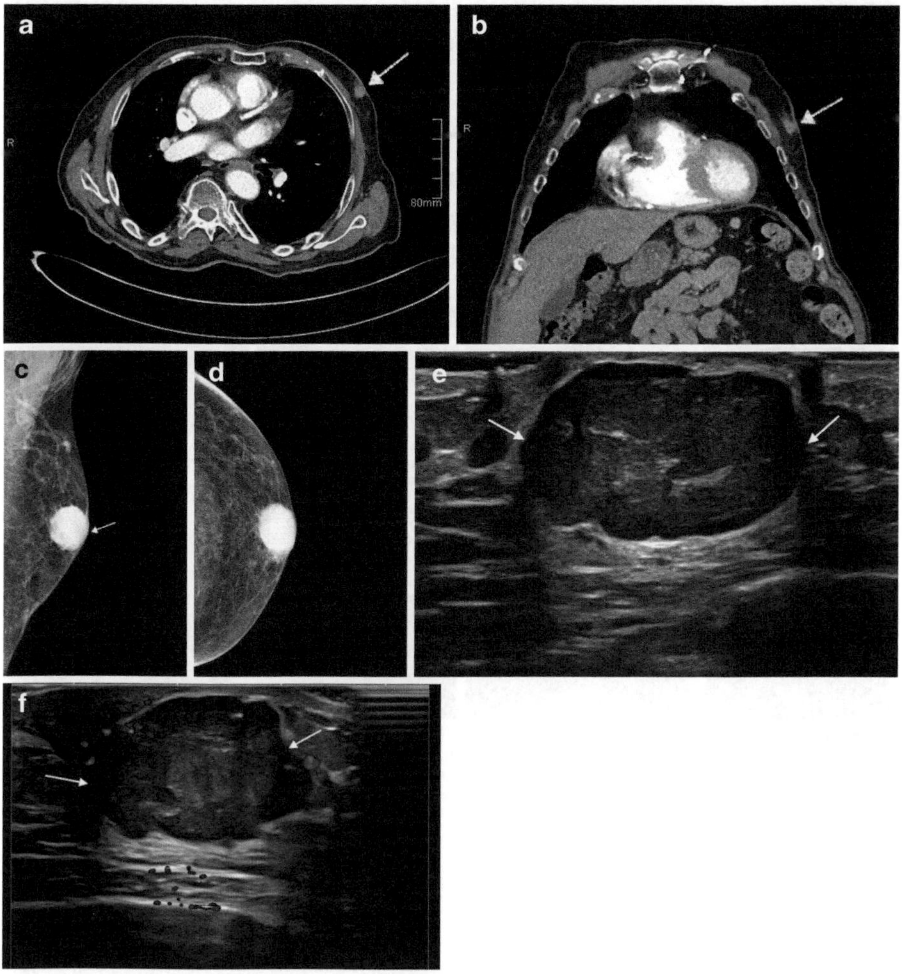

Fig. 4.4 Male breast cancer. Axial CT chest without IV contrast (**a**), coronal view (**b**), right breast mammography MLO view (**c**), CC view (**d**), grayscale ultrasound (**e**), and color Doppler ultrasound (**f**). The chest CT in a male patient revealed a soft tissue irregular shape enhancing mass in the left retroareolar region (arrow). Left breast two-view mammography demonstrates a dense mass with an angular margin in the left retro nipple (arrow). The ultrasound examination confirmed a hypoechoic, solid mass with some vascularity on color Doppler. The mass underwent an ultrasound-guided biopsy and yielded a grade 2 invasive breast cancer with micropapillary features that was ER and PR positive and HER2 negative

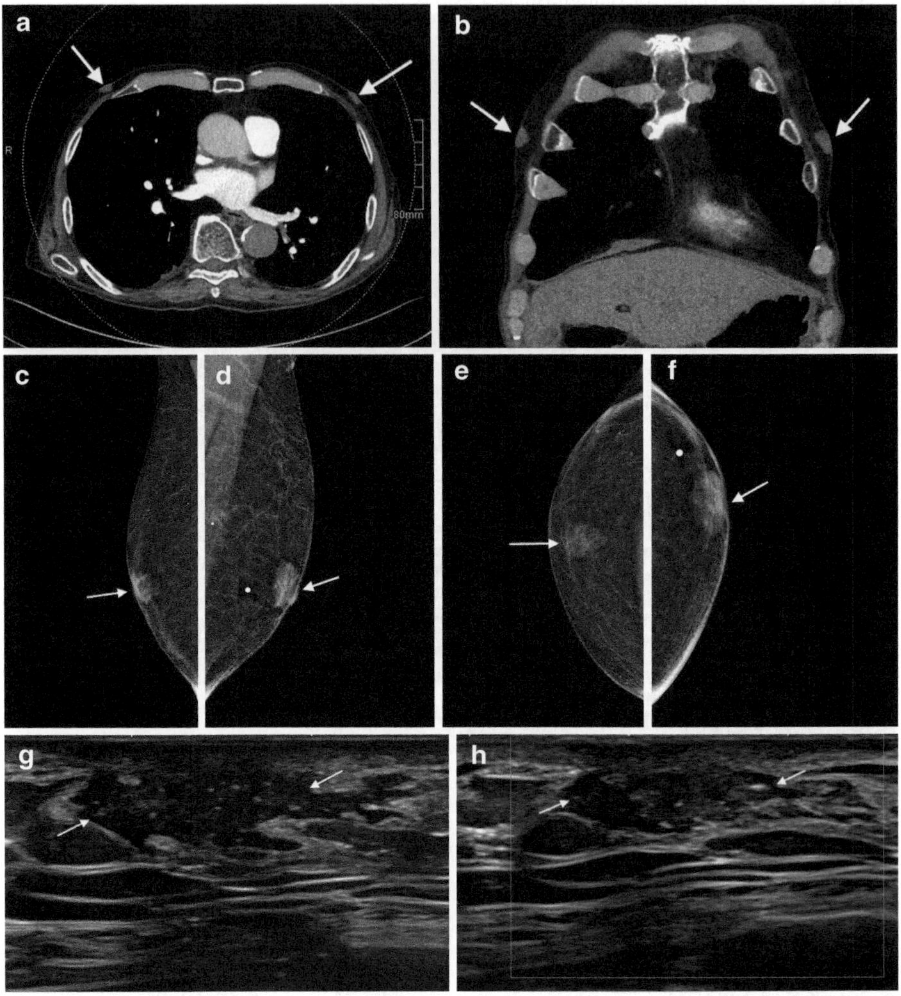

Fig. 4.5 Bilateral nodular gynecomastia. Axial CT chest without IV contrast (**a**), coronal view (**b**), bilateral breast mammography MLO view (**c, d**), CC view (**e, f**), grayscale ultrasound (**g**), and color Doppler ultrasound (**h**). The chest CT in a male patient revealed bilateral small, retro nipple, central, subjectively with no significant enhancing, symmetric soft tissue lesions (arrows). Bilateral breast two-view mammography demonstrates symmetric retro nipple nodular densities (arrows). The patient felt a lump in the left breast, which was marked on the skin with a BB marker. The ultrasound examination confirmed a hypoechoic, flame-shaped, non-mass lesion with no detectable vascularity on color Doppler. The findings reported nodular gynecomastia, and BI-RADS 2 was given with a recommendation for clinical follow-up. Nodular gynecomastia is a type of benign male breast enlargement along with dendritic and diffuse types. It can appear as a dense, palpable, button-shaped mass beneath the nipple

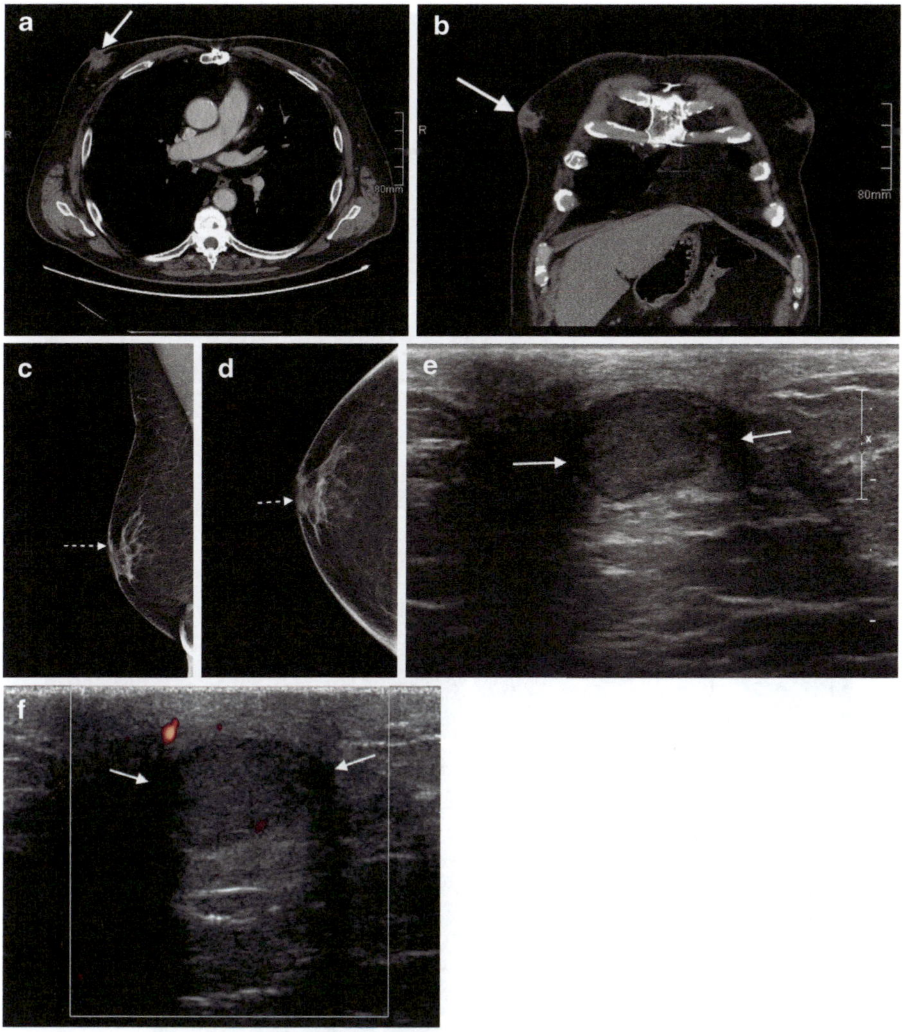

Fig. 4.6 Retroareolar abscess of male breast. Axial chest CT scan with IV contrast (**a**), coronal view (**b**), mammography MLO view (**c**), mammography CC view (**d**), grayscale ultrasound (**e**), and color Doppler ultrasound (**f**). Chest CT scan of a male patient at the level of nipples shows bilateral increased fibroglandular tissue suggestive of gynecomastia. In the right breast, retro nipple, oval fluid density mass with peripheral thin rim enhancement (solid arrow) is noted, associated with the patient's clinical signs of inflammation. Mammogram, two views, demonstrated increased central fibroglandular tissue suggestive of gynecomastia with mild central skin thickening, consistent with inflammation (dashed arrow). Ultrasound showed a retroareolar oval hypoechoic mass with posterior through transmission, increased peripheral hyper-echogenicity, and vascularity, suggestive of inflammatory changes. The mass underwent an ultrasound-guided fine-needle aspiration and collapsed; the fluid was sent for cytology and microbiology tests, which yielded benign breast parenchyma with acute, chronic inflammation and abscess. No fungal or microbacterial organisms were identified on Giemsa, Gram, or Ziehl-Neelsen stains. Clinically, Zuska's disease, subareolar breast abscess (SBA) of the male breast, which is a rare recurrent infectious disease of the breast in males, was suggested

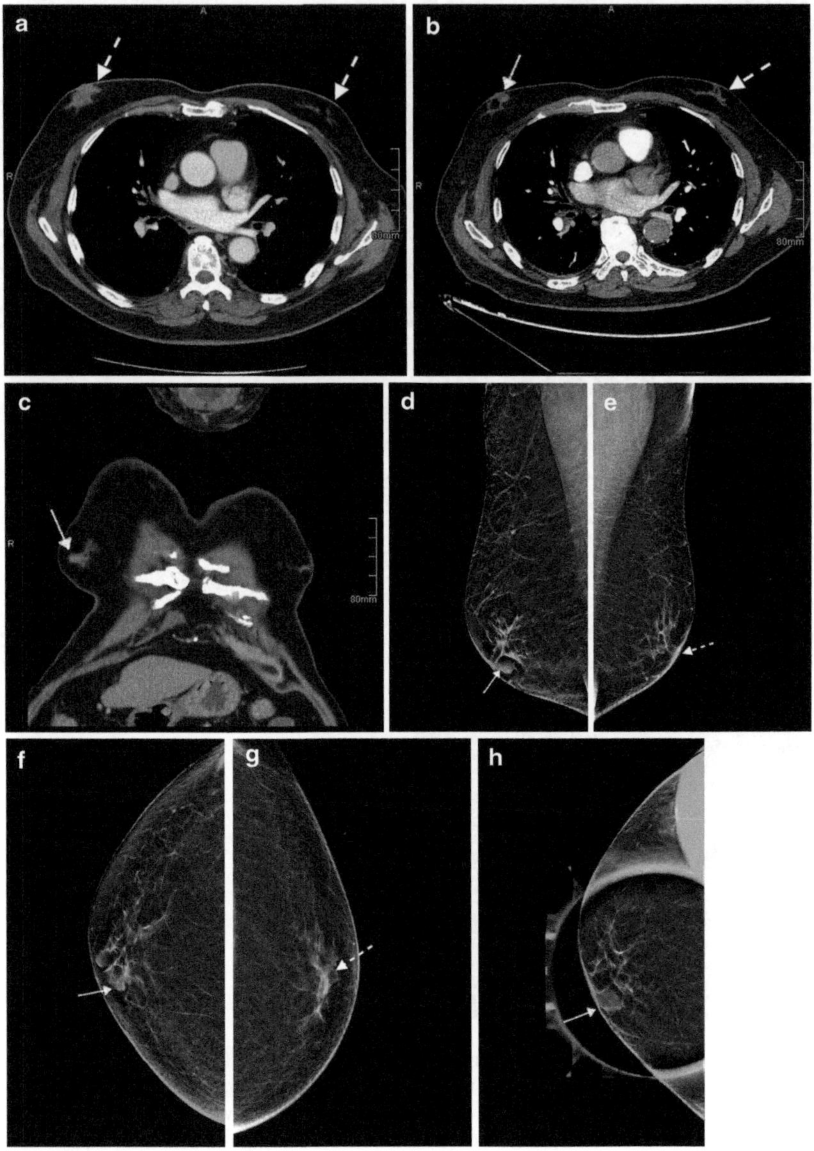

Fig. 4.7 Papillary breast carcinoma of male breast. Axial chest CT scan with IV contrast (**a, b**), coronal view (**c**), mammography MLO view (**d, e**), mammography CC view (**f, g**), mammography focal spot view (**h**), grayscale ultrasound (**i**), and color Doppler ultrasound (**j**). Chest CT scan of a male patient at the level of the nipple shows bilateral, retro nipple, asymmetrically increased fibroglandular tissue, more on the right side, suggestive of gynecomastia (dashed arrow). Additionally, at the lower level, in the right lower inner breast, there is a nodular soft tissue mass (solid arrow). A bilateral two-view mammogram demonstrates bilateral gynecomastia with a right lower inner retro nipple isodense mass (solid arrow). Ultrasound showed a retroareolar, roundish, vascular, hypoechoic, solid mass with some internal cystic components. The mass underwent an ultrasound-guided core needle biopsy, which yielded papillary carcinoma of the male breast, which is rare, slow-growing, with a better prognosis than invasive ductal carcinoma

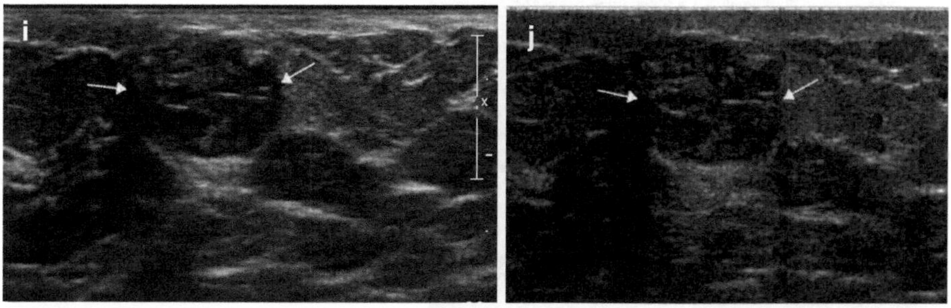

Fig. 4.7 (continued)

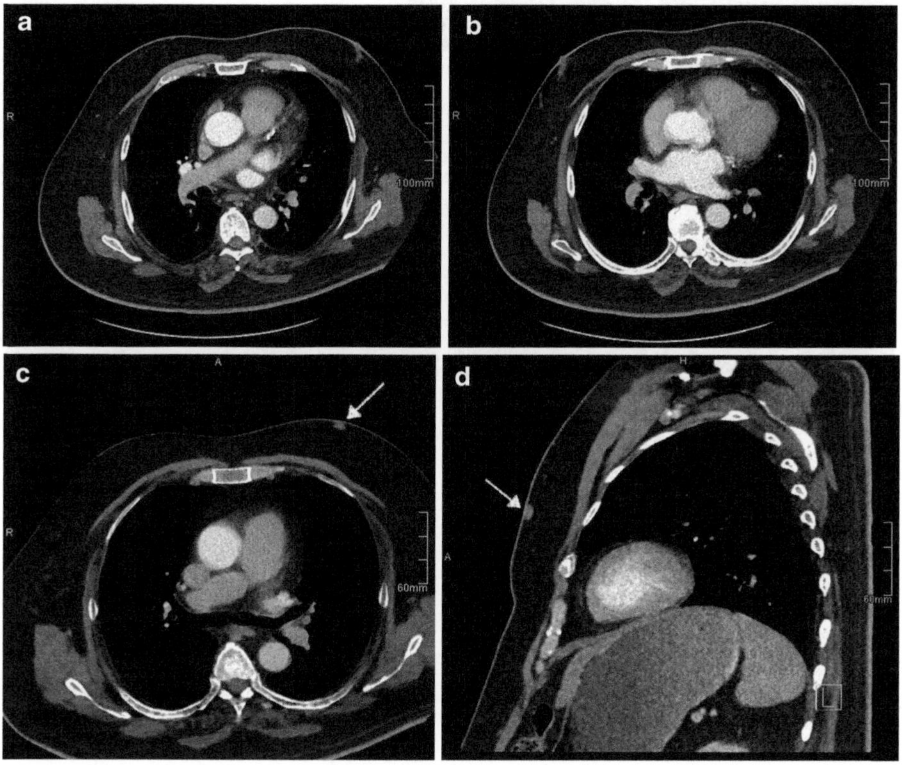

Fig. 4.8 Hemangioma in male breast. Axial chest CT scan with IV contrast at left retro nipple level (**a**), at right retro nipple level (**b**), at the level of a palpable concern (**c**), chest CT scan sagittal view (**d**), mammography MLO view (**e**), mammography CC view (**f**), grayscale ultrasound (**g**), and color Doppler ultrasound (**h**). Chest CT scan of a male patient at the level of nipples shows bilateral small gynecomastia. In the central inner left breast, a superficial, oval-shaped soft tissue mass with subtle enhancement (arrow) is noted, consistent with the patient's clinical concern of a lump. On mammogram, two views, a slight increase in retro nipple fibroglandular tissue suggestive of mild gynecomastia was noted. Additionally, consistent with the patient's clinical concern of a lump, BB markers on the skin, a superficially located, oval, circumscribed mass without associated calcification or distortion is noted (arrow). Ultrasound demonstrated a subcutaneous oval mass with internal cystic components and mild vascularity on color Doppler. The mass underwent an ultrasound-guided biopsy, which yielded a benign hemangioma. Male hemangioma is an uncommon, benign vascular tumor that typically presents as a palpable mass. A biopsy is required for a definitive diagnosis

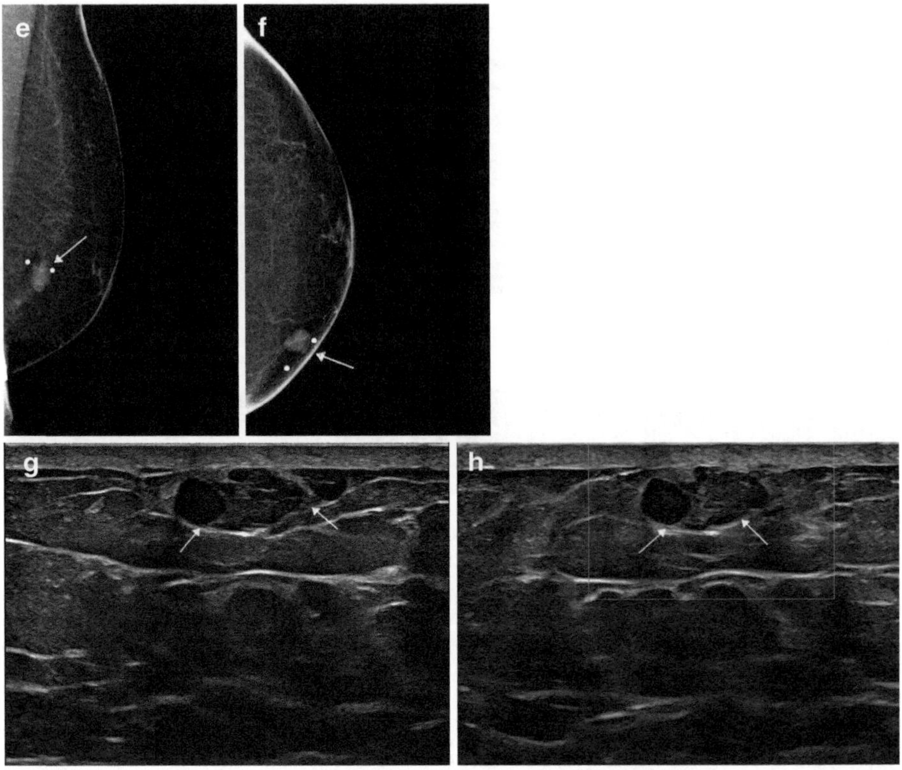

Fig. 4.8 (continued)

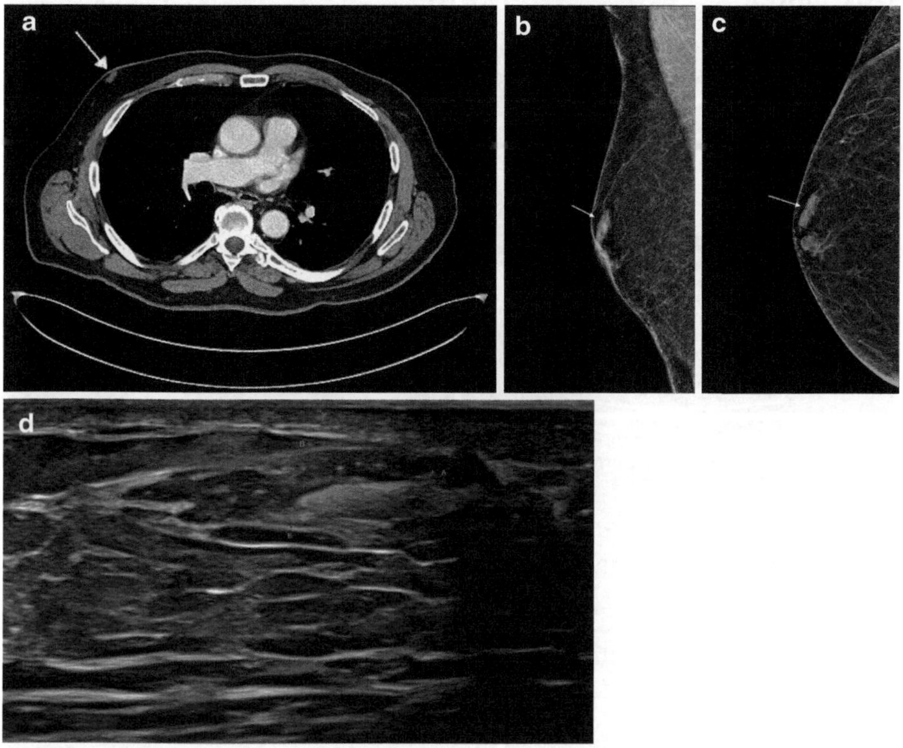

Fig. 4.9 Lymphoma in male breast. Axial chest CT scan with IV contrast (**a**), mammography MLO view (**b**), CC view (**c**), and ultrasound grayscale (**d**). A male patient with a history of multiple cancers including squamous cell carcinoma of the anal canal, marginal zone lymphoma, prostate cancer, and papillary left renal carcinoma underwent a follow-up chest CT scan. The CT scan revealed a new elongated eccentric soft tissue mass with minimally enhancement in his right upper breast (arrow). The mammogram showed a mass in the right upper outer quadrant without associated calcifications. In the ultrasound, the corresponding lesion was identified at the 10 o'clock position as an elongated, slightly heterogeneous, hypovascular solid mass. An ultrasound-guided core needle biopsy confirmed the diagnosis of low-grade lymphoma

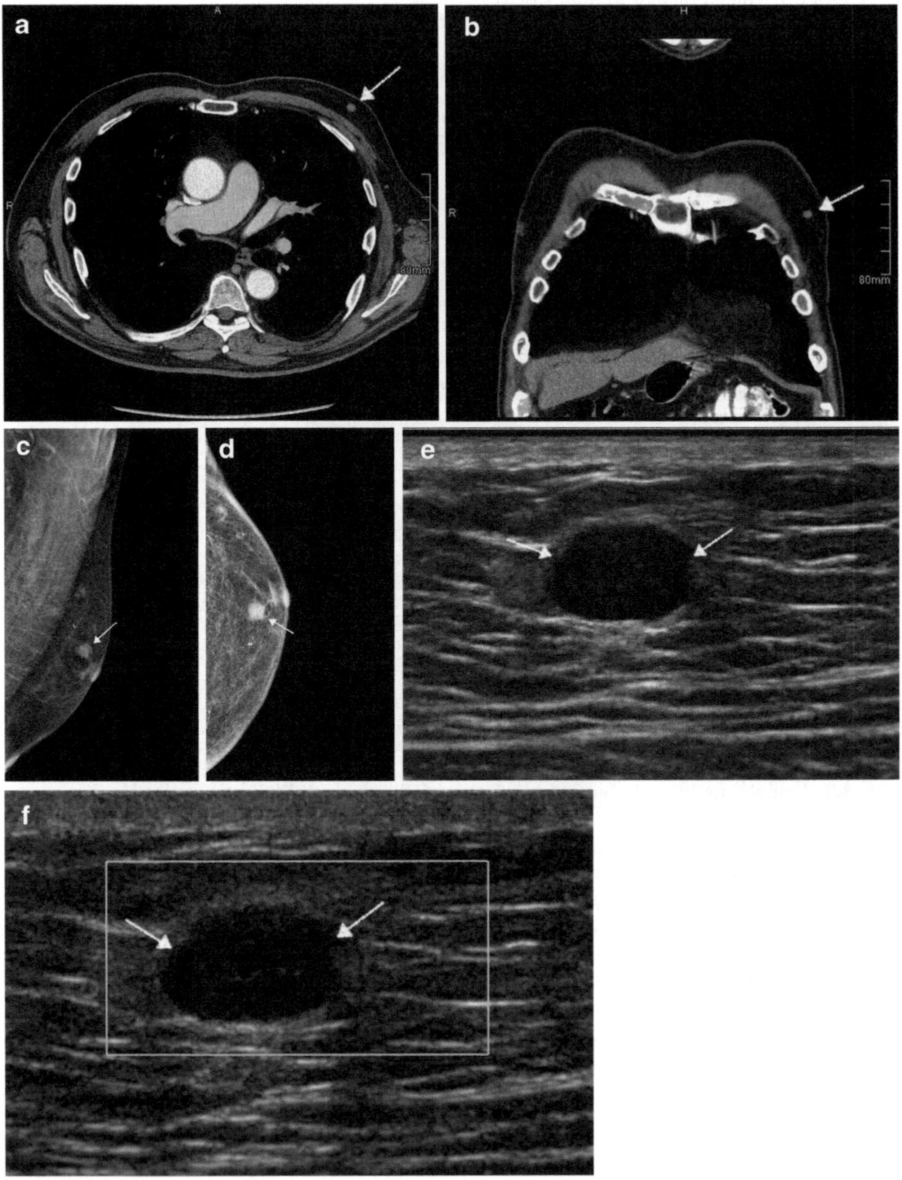

Fig. 4.10 Metastasis of Melanoma in male breast. Axial chest CT scan with IV contrast (**a**), coronal view (**b**), mammography MLO view (**c**), mammography CC view (**d**), grayscale ultrasound (**e**), and color Doppler ultrasound (**f**). Chest CT scan of a male patient shows a circumscribed, enhancing, subcentimeter mass in the left central breast (solid arrow). Mammogram demonstrates a well-circumscribed mass in the left upper central breast (arrow). On ultrasound, a significantly hypoechoic, hypovascular solid mass with posterior through transmission was noted. The mass underwent an ultrasound-guided core needle biopsy, which yielded a melanoma metastasis. The patient had a history of extremity melanoma. In men with a history of melanoma who develop a new breast lump, metastasis of melanoma is uncommon but probable and necessitates a high index of suspicion

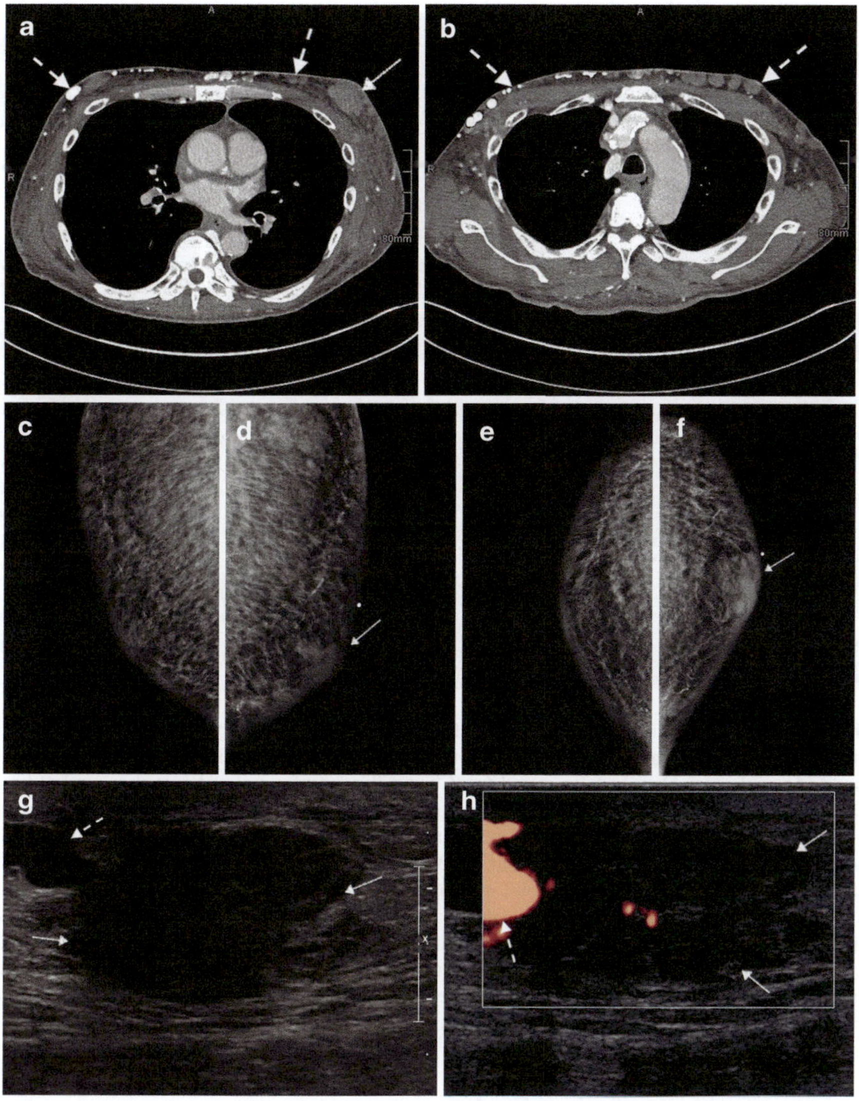

Fig. 4.11 Gynecomastia with PASH. Axial chest CT scan with IV contrast (**a, b**), mammography MLO view (**c, d**), mammography CC view (**e, f**), grayscale ultrasound (**g**), and color Doppler ultrasound (**h**). Chest CT scan of a male patient shows bilateral breast edema, superficial dilated vessels (dashed arrows), and a left retro nipple flame-shaped soft tissue mass (solid arrow). Bilateral mammogram was performed demonstrating generalized skin thickening, trabecular thickening and signs of breast edema. Additionally, consistent with the patient's clinical concern of a lump and BB marker on the skin in the left central breast, a mass with an indistinct border in the left retro nipple region was noted (solid arrow). On ultrasound, a significantly hypoechoic, solid mass with internal cystic components and vascularity was seen. Adjacent to the mass, dilated vascular structures were also identified (dashed arrow). The patient had a history of longstanding end-stage renal disease on dialysis, which could explain bilateral generalized significant breast edema. The left retro nipple mass underwent an ultrasound-guided core needle biopsy, which yielded gynecomastia with benign breast tissue with pseudoangiomatous stromal hyperplasia (PASH) as well as usual hyperplasia. The pathology results were considered concordant, and clinical follow-up was suggested

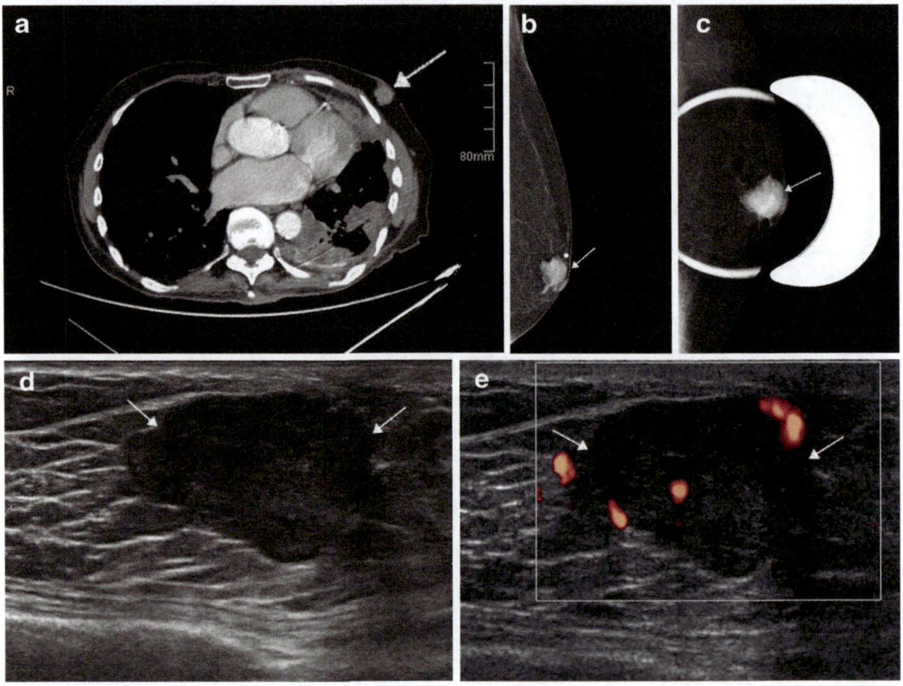

Fig. 4.12 Invasive carcinoma with papillary features in male breast. Axial chest CT scan with IV contrast (**a**), mammography MLO view and focal compression spot view (**b, c**), grayscale ultrasound (**d**), and color Doppler ultrasound (**e**). Chest CT scan of a male patient shows a left breast retro nipple, lobulated, enhancing soft tissue mass (arrow). Additionally, there are some peripheral lung opacities related to the patient's known history of lung cancer. Mammogram corresponding to the patient's clinical concern of a lump and BB marker on the skin in the left central breast demonstrates a dense lobulated mass (arrow) with underlying increased fibroglandular tissue (gynecomastia). On ultrasound, a hypoechoic, solid mass with internal cystic components and increased vascularity was seen. The mass underwent an ultrasound-guided core needle biopsy, which yielded invasive carcinoma with papillary features. In immunohistochemistry, the tumor was ER, PR, and Gata3 diffusely positive, p63 and msm negative, and Napsin and TTF1 negative. The overall morphology and immunoprofile were more consistent with a breast primary cancer in a male patient

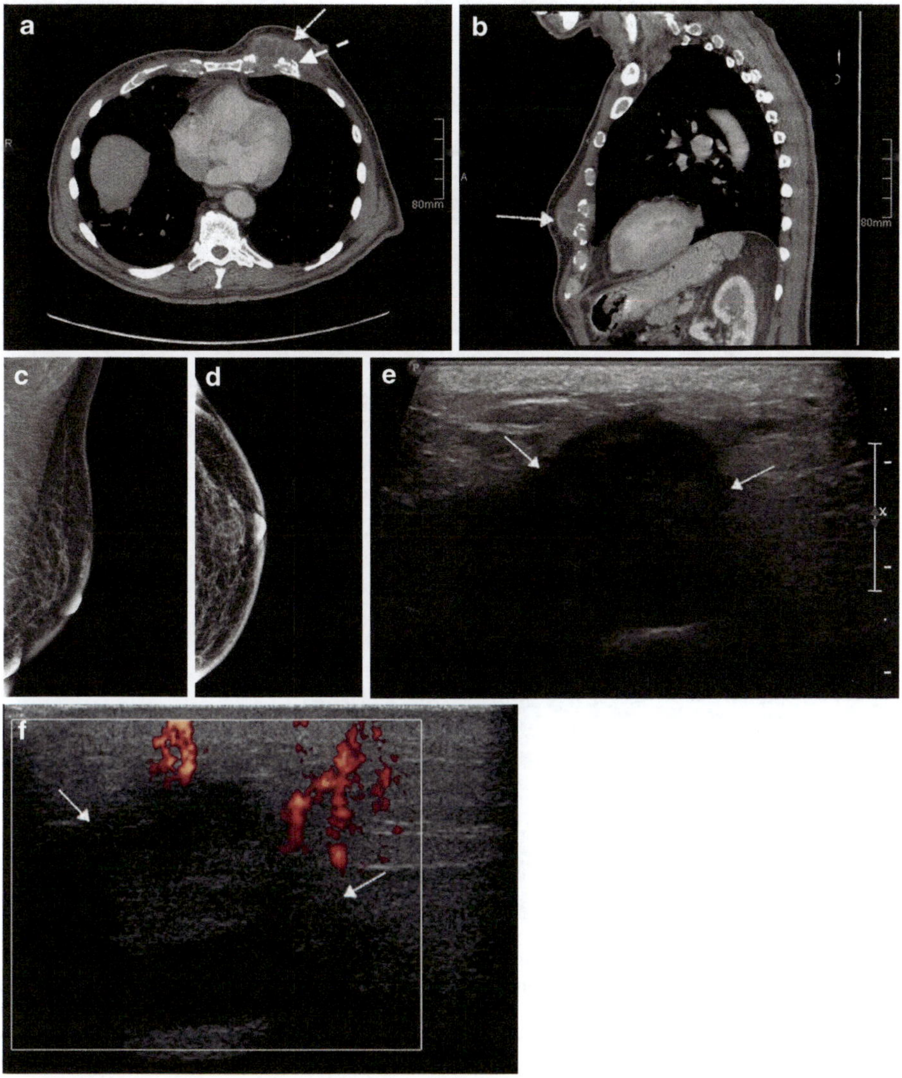

Fig. 4.13 Cholangiocarcinoma metastasis to chest wall presenting as a breast mass. Axial chest CT scan with IV contrast (**a**), sagittal chest CT scan (**b**), mammography MLO view (**c**), CC view (**d**), grayscale ultrasound (**e**), and color Doppler ultrasound (**f**). Chest CT scan of a male patient shows a deeply located soft tissue mass with peripheral rim enhancement and central low density (solid arrow) in the left breast associated with underlying rib destruction (dashed arrow). The mammogram did not include the deeply located mass. Ultrasound demonstrated a hypoechoic, solid mass with some peripheral vascularity. The posterior border of the mass was poorly visualized and blended with the chest wall. The mass underwent an ultrasound-guided core needle biopsy, which yielded well to moderately differentiated adenocarcinoma with no benign glandular breast tissue. Tumor cells were positive for K7 and CDX2 and negative for Napsin A, GATA3, ER, AR, PSA, and WT. The findings overall suggested a cholangiocarcinoma metastasis. The patient had a known advanced biliary cholangiocarcinoma

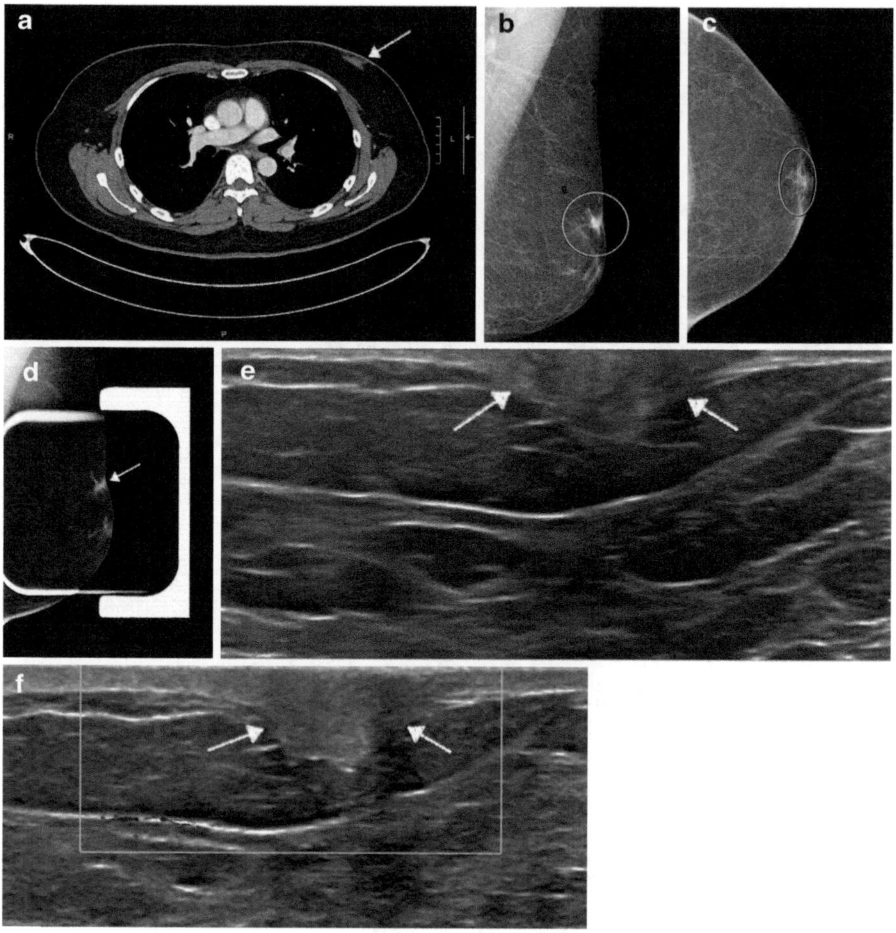

Fig. 4.14 Invasive male breast carcinoma with neuroendocrine differentiation. Axial chest CT scan with IV contrast (**a**), mammography MLO view (**b**), CC view (**c**), focal compression spot view (**d**), grayscale ultrasound (**e**), and color Doppler ultrasound (**f**). Chest CT scan of a male patient shows a superficial, eccentric, irregular shaped soft tissue mass in the upper central left breast (arrow). The mammogram shows an irregular dense subdermal mass in the left upper central breast (circle and arrow), ultrasound examination showed a heterogeneous, hyperechoic, subdermal, hypovascular solid mass. An ultrasound-guided core needle biopsy was performed, which confirmed the presence of invasive male breast carcinoma with neuroendocrine differentiation. Immunohistochemistry results indicated that the tumor cells were diffusely and strongly positive for estrogen receptor (ER) and GATA3, with isolated cells expressing mammaglobin. Neuroendocrine differentiation in breast carcinoma is not uncommon. According to the 2019 edition of the WHO classification of tumors, invasive breast carcinoma with neuroendocrine differentiation is considered a morphological variant of invasive carcinoma of no special type for treatment purposes

References

1. Dershaw DD. Imaging the male breast. Semin Roentgenol. 2010;45(3):181–8.
2. O'Connor DJ, Menes TS. Imaging of the male breast. Clin Radiol. 2019;74(2):98–108.
3. Iuanow E, Kettler M, Slanetz PJ. Male breast disease: a review with radiologic-pathologic correlation. Radiographics. 2011;31(3):795–817.
4. Evans GF, Anthony T, Turnage RH, Schumpert TD, Levy KR, Amirkhan RH. The radiologic evaluation of male breast disease. Radiographics. 2001;21(4):993–1005.
5. Yang WT, Whitman GJ, Yuen EH, Tse GM, Stelling CB. Sonographic, mammographic, and CT features of male breast cancer. AJR Am J Roentgenol. 2001;176(2):413–8.
6. Johnson RE, Murad MH. Gynecomastia: pathophysiology, evaluation, and management. Mayo Clin Proc. 2009;84(11):1010–5.
7. Vassiou K, Tsikouras P, Tsapaki V. Gynecomastia: Imaging findings with emphasis on MRI, CT, and PET/CT. Clin Imaging. 2010;34(5):345–9.
8. Yalaza M, Inan A, Bozer M. Male breast cancer. J Breast Health. 2016;12(1):1–8.
9. Giordano SH. Breast cancer in men. N Engl J Med. 2018;378(24):2311–20.

Chapter 5
Breast Reconstruction and Augmentation: Incidental Findings on Chest CT

Introduction

As the incidence of breast cancer increases and surgical procedures advance, breast reconstruction following mastectomy is becoming more common. Radiologic imaging is essential for assessing both normal postoperative changes and complications. The two main reconstruction techniques are implant-based reconstruction, which uses silicone or saline prostheses, frequently with acellular dermal matrix support, and autologous tissue reconstruction, which uses the patient's own tissue (e.g., DIEP, TRAM, latissimus dorsi flaps). Although autologous reconstructions typically result in a neobreast with a more natural contour and softness, there is a wide range of anticipated imaging appearances and possible surgical complications, including fat necrosis, seroma, or vascular impairment. The potential issues include capsular contracture, implant intra and extra capsular rupture, and rare disorders such as breast implant-associated large cell lymphoma (BIA-ALCL). Accurately interpreting and distinguishing benign postsurgical alterations from pathologies, specifically recurrence, requires an understanding of these entities [1–3].

Although less frequently used than MRI or ultrasound in routine postoperative evaluation, CT imaging of the reconstructed breast offers useful cross-sectional detail that can help define flap integrity, detect fluid collections, and evaluate donor site complications like abdominal wall defects or hernias. CT scan can depict the intricate architecture of autologous flaps with muscle, subcutaneous fat, and skin. Expected postoperative changes include seromas and soft tissue edema. Flap necrosis and abscesses are examples of complications that manifest as focal low-attenuation areas with rim enhancement or, if infected, gas. Although CT can display implant location, peri-implant fluid, or gross extracapsular silicone in the event of rupture in implant reconstructions, MRI is preferable for comprehensive implant evaluation. Diagnostic precision is increased by familiarity with the typical postoperative CT spectrum and associated complications [3–5].

A. Alikhassi, *Atlas of Breast Lesions on Chest Computed Tomography*,
https://doi.org/10.1007/978-3-032-22791-1_5

When assessing the soft tissue composition, vascular pedicles in autologous flaps, and the possible recurrence of reconstructed breasts, MRI remains the preferred method. The selection of imaging modalities and knowledge of the type of reconstruction have a major impact on the accuracy of diagnosis and differentiation of recurrence or remnant cancer from benign postoperative changes [1, 6, 7]. Mammography and ultrasound are also useful tools for imaging the reconstructed breast. Although ultrasound is excellent for assessing superficial collections (seromas, hematomas), guiding biopsies, and describing focal masses, its use may be restricted in deep flaps or behind implants. Mammography shows fat-containing autologous flaps or calcifications associated with fat necrosis or prior therapy. Mammography is not usually performed after reconstruction unless for symptomatic evaluation or screening of residual breast tissue.

Overall, the greatest results are obtained with a multimodality imaging strategy customized to the type of reconstruction and the clinical concern [2, 4, 8].

Figures 5.1, 5.2, 5.3, 5.4, 5.5, 5.6, 5.7, 5.8, 5.9, and 5.10 illustrate cases involving the use of chest CT scans in breast reconstruction/augmentation.

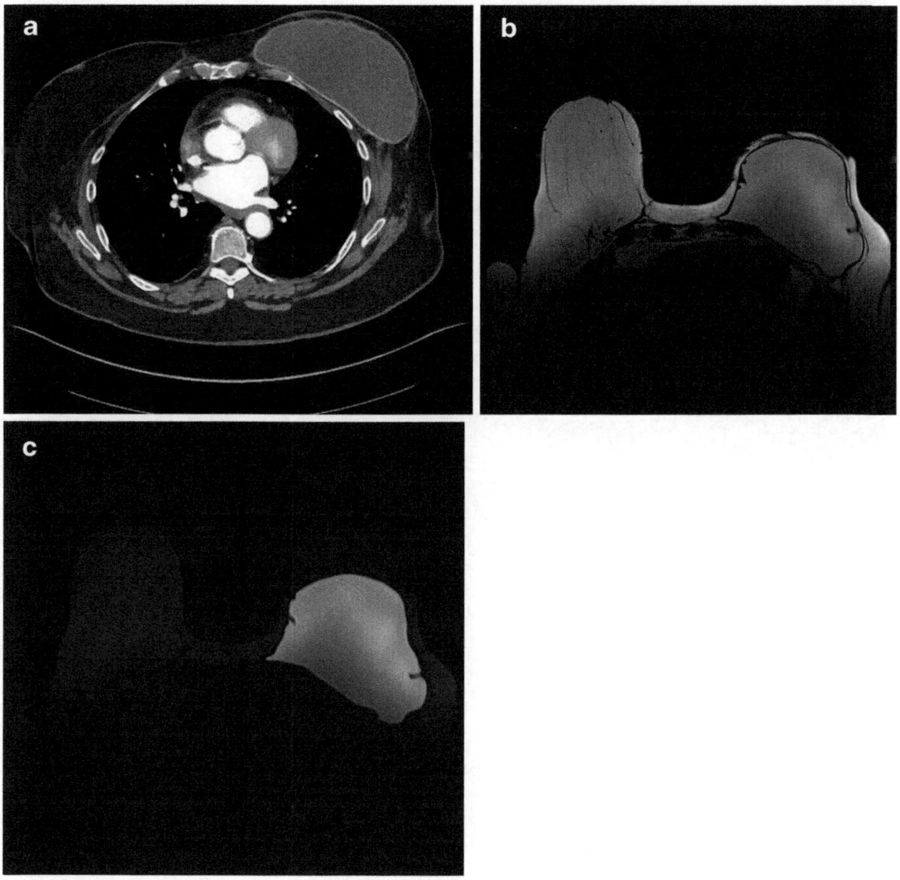

Fig. 5.1 Reconstructed breasts. Chest CT scan with contrast axial view (**a**), MRI T1-weighted axial view (**b**), and MRI silicone-specific view (**c**) of a patient who has undergone bilateral breast mastectomy and reconstruction. The chest CT scan illustrates the right breast with autologous flap reconstruction, displaying entirely fatty tissue, and the left breast with silicone implant reconstruction. On the MRI, utilizing the implant integrity protocol, the flap-reconstructed right breast appears entirely fatty, while the left breast silicone implant remains intact

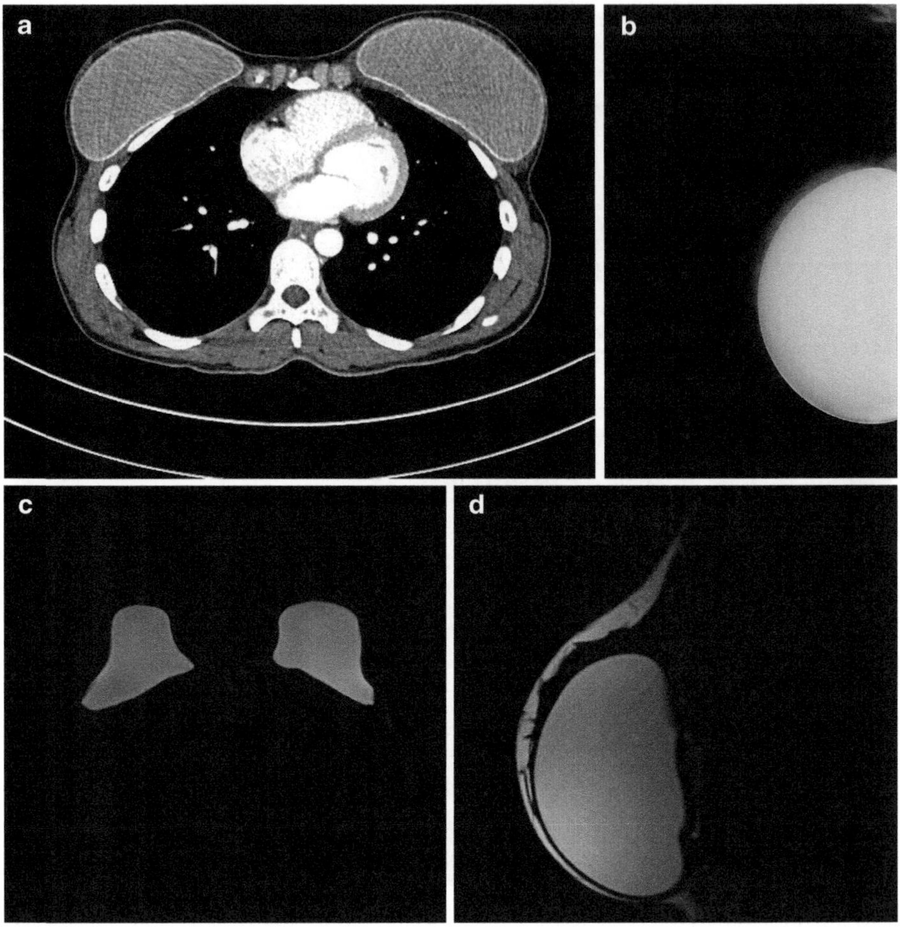

Fig. 5.2 Intact silicone implant. Chest CT scan with contrast axial view (**a**), right breast CC view mammography (**b**), MRI silicone-specific sequence axial view (**c**), and MRI silicone-specific sequence sagittal view (**d**) images demonstrate intact retropectoral silicone implants

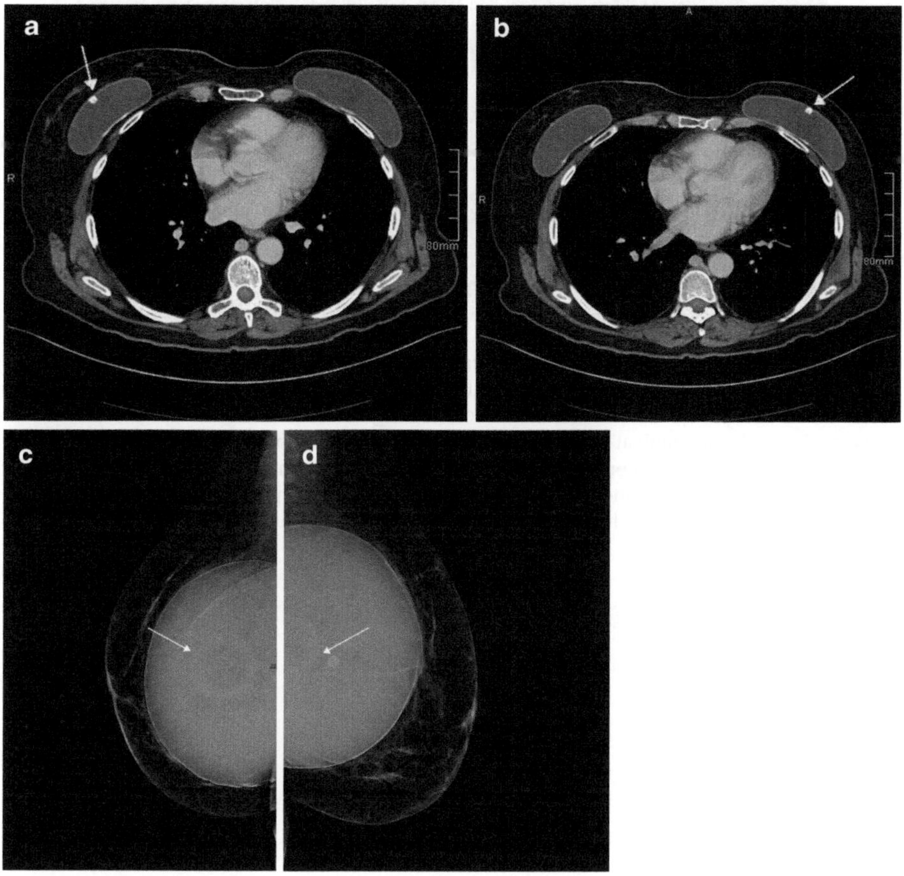

Fig. 5.3 Saline implant. Chest CT scan axial view (**a**, **b**) and bilateral mammography MLO view (**c**, **d**) images demonstrate typical intact bilateral normal saline implant. Notably, saline implants have valves (arrow) that help differentiate them from silicone implants on a CT scan. Saline implants typically display fluid density on a CT scan

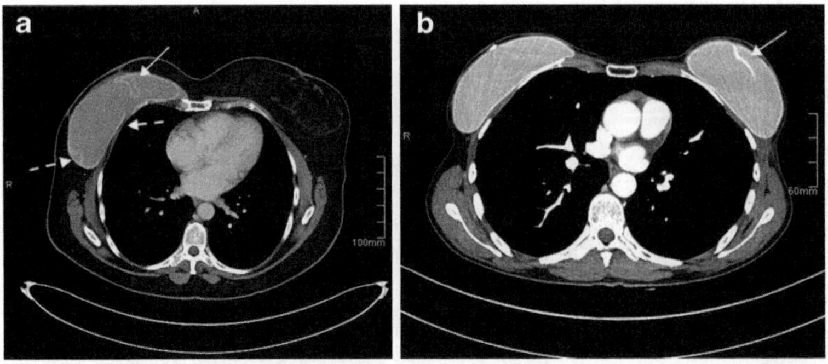

Fig. 5.4 Implant fold or rupture. Chest CT scan axial view (**a**, **b**). The chest CT scan in image **a** revealed signs of an intracapsular implant rupture, characterized by the presence of linguine signs (solid arrow) and subcapsular lines (dashed arrows). Image **b** shows a normal implant fold. Normal radial folds in a breast implant are normal invaginations of the implant shell, typically characterized by a straight, thick, and short appearance extending to the implant surface (arrow). Intracapsular ruptures are characterized by the rupture of the implant shell with an intact fibrous capsule that can present with linguine signs with multiple curvilinear, low-signal-intensity lines within the silicone gel or subcapsular lines

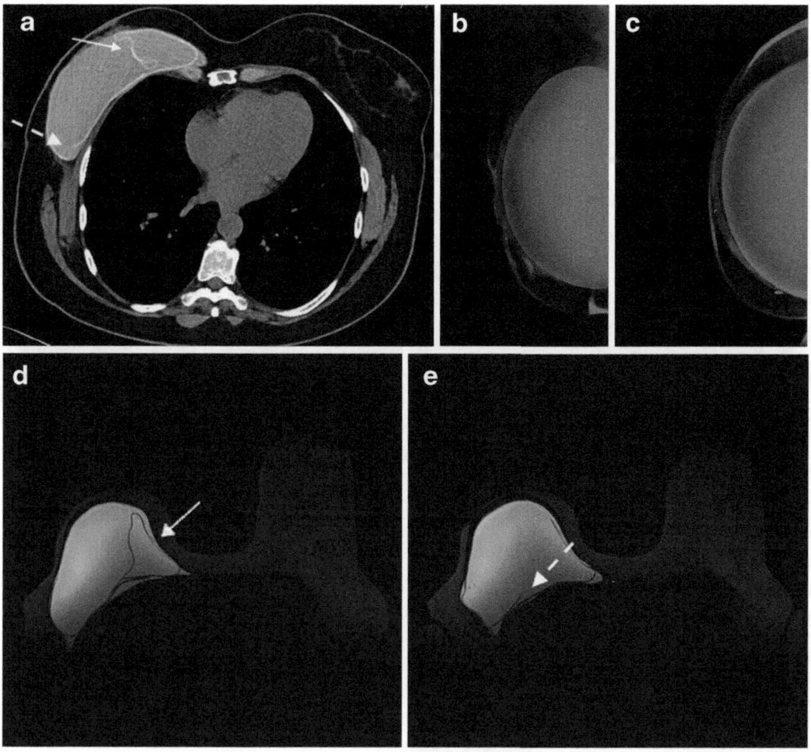

Fig. 5.5 Implant intracapsular rupture. Chest CT scan axial view (**a**), mammography MLO view (**b**), CC view (**c**), and MRI silicone-specific axial view (**d, e**) of a woman with a history of right breast skin-sparing mastectomy and implant reconstruction revealed signs of an intracapsular implant rupture, characterized by the presence of a subcapsular line (dashed arrow) and linguine signs (solid arrows) in both the CT scan and MRI. No significant abnormalities were appreciated in the mammography images

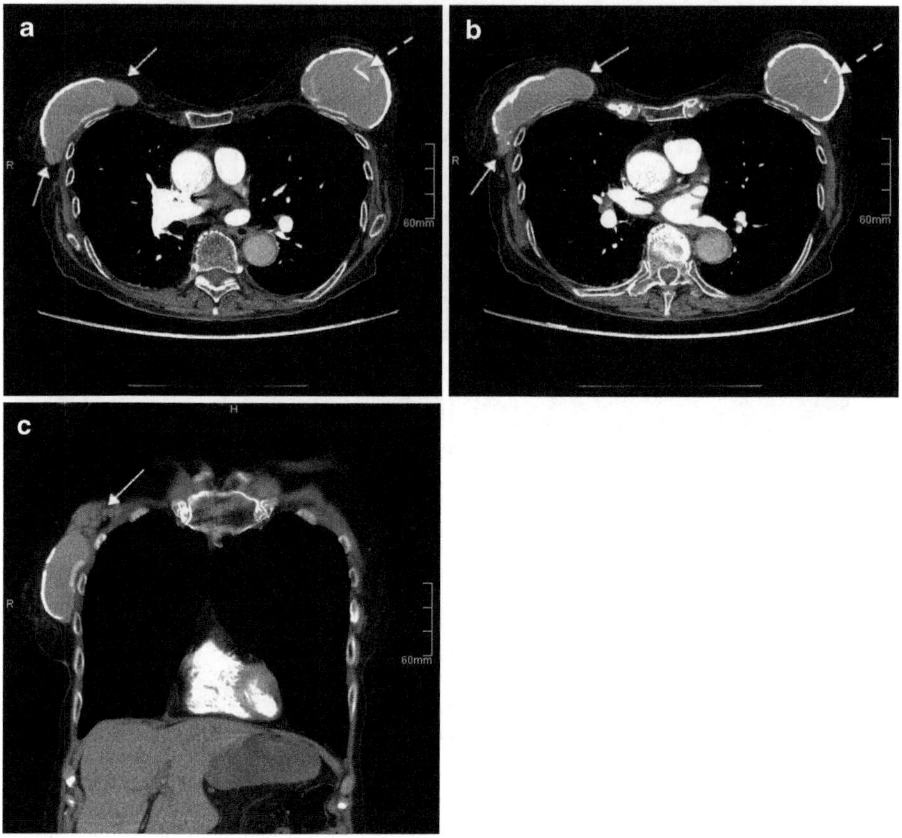

Fig. 5.6 Implant extracapsular rupture. Chest CT scan axial view (**a, b**) and coronal view (**c**) show right implant capsular calcification, capsular defect and protrusion of silicone outside the implant border (solid arrows), favoring implant extracapsular rupture. In the left implant, capsular calcification, a subtle subcapsular line in medial side suggestive of intracapsular rupture and a normal implant fold (dashed arrow) are noted

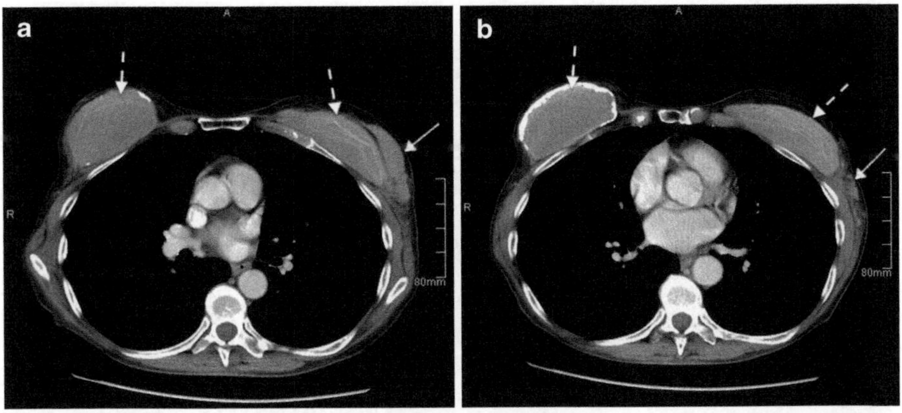

Fig. 5.7 Implant intra- and extracapsular rupture. Chest CT scan axial view (**a, b**) illustrates capsular calcification around the right implant and bilateral subcapsular lines (dashed arrows), which suggest an intracapsular rupture of the implants. Additionally, on the left side, there are defects in the capsule and multiple silicone accumulations outside the implant capsule, indicating an extracapsular rupture (solid arrow)

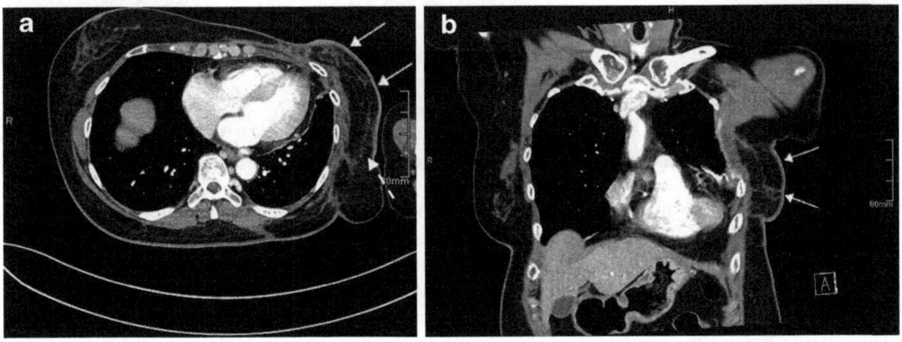

Fig. 5.8 Autologous flap reconstruction. Chest CT scan axial view (**a**) and coronal view (**b**) of a woman with a history of left breast cancer and mastectomy illustrates signs of autologous flap reconstruction (solid arrow). A reconstructed breast often appears predominantly fatty and potentially shows muscle remnants or vascular pedicles. Potential complications, such as fat necrosis or infection, should be sought in all cases. A contact line (dashed arrow) at the junction of residual subcutaneous fat and implanted flap adipose tissue is characteristic

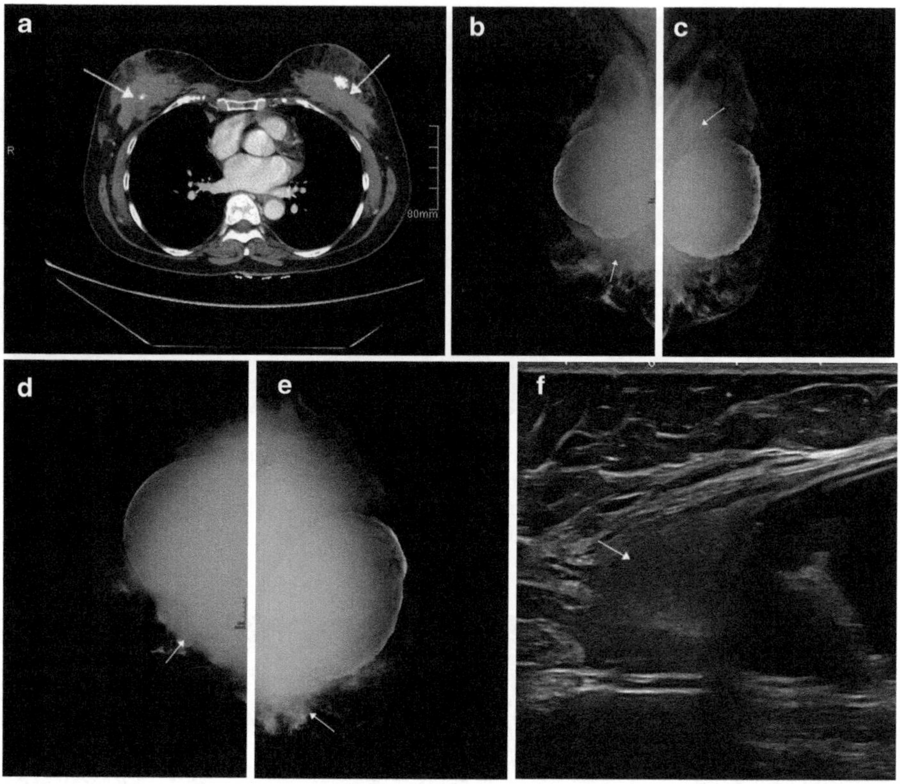

Fig. 5.9 Free silicone injection. Chest CT scan axial view (**a**), bilateral mammography MLO views (**b, c**), CC views (**d, e**), and grayscale ultrasound (**f**) of a woman with a history of bilateral free silicone injection and subsequent silicone implant augmentation. The CT image shows dense shapeless deposits in the breast with calcifications; the implants were not included in this CT level. Bilateral mammography also shows a retroglandular silicone implant with a calcified capsule and dense tissue behind the implants, corresponding to the history of remote free silicone injection (arrow). Ultrasound shows hyperechoic materials with posterior shadowing suggestive of snowstorm appearance surrounding the implant. The "snowstorm" appearance is a characteristic ultrasound finding indicating the presence of free silicone in breast (injection or ruptured implants). Free silicone breast injections are an alternative form of breast augmentation to breast implants and are banned in North America. Characteristic imaging results from free silicone injection of the breast include high-attenuation material on mammography, a silicone signal with varied granulomatous reactivity on MRI, and an echogenic "snowstorm" artifact on ultrasound. Correlation between modalities is crucial, as these alterations can mask normal breast architecture and significantly limit the detection of malignancy. Complications include silicone migration, lymph node involvement, and persistent inflammation

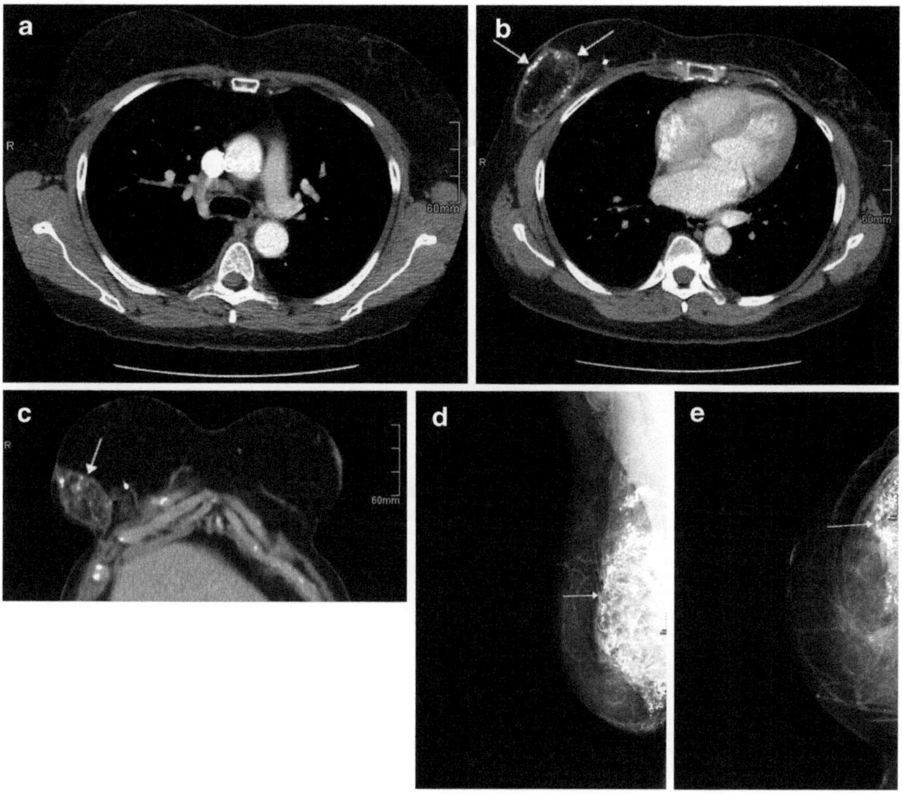

Fig. 5.10 Flap reconstruction with fat necrosis. Chest CT scan axial view (**a, b**), coronal view (**c**), right mammography MLO view (**d**), and CC view (**e**) of a woman with a history of right lumpectomy, axillary dissection, and radiation, followed by mastectomy, TRAM flap reconstruction, and left breast reduction surgery. The CT image shows a predominantly fatty reconstructed breast with a peripherally calcified, fat-containing mass (arrow) in the lateral deep breast, which is typical of fat necrosis. Right breast mammography findings parallel the chest CT scan finding with a predominantly reconstructed breast and deeply located dystrophic calcifications (arrow) suggestive of fat necrosis. A typical and anticipated complication of autologous breast reconstruction is fat necrosis, caused by adipose tissue ischemia and subsequent fibrotic and inflammatory evolution of the fatty tissue. Its appearance on imaging is highly variable and modality dependent. For a precise diagnosis and suitable treatment, correlation with surgical history, temporal evolution, and multimodality imaging is crucial

References

1. American College of Radiology. ACR Appropriateness Criteria→ imaging after mastectomy and breast reconstruction. J Am Coll Radiol 2020;17(11S):S410-S420.
2. Kanavou T, Vasileiou G, Vryonidou A, et al. Imaging of the reconstructed breast: a multimodality approach. Insights Imaging. 2023;14(1):176.
3. Vasileiou G, Kanavou T, Kapsoritakis A, et al. Multimodality imaging of breast reconstruction: normal appearances and complications. Cancer Imaging. 2024;24(1):12.

4. Lee SH, Kim EK, Kim MJ. CT appearance of breast reconstruction and postoperative complications. Radiographics. 2012;32(5):1369–86.
5. Srinivasa DR, Clemens MW, Qi J, et al. Imaging and donor-site complications following autologous breast reconstruction. Plast Reconstr Surg. 2021;147(5):1019–30.
6. Cher DJ, Conwell JM, Mandel JS. MRI of the reconstructed breast: distinguishing benign postoperative findings from malignancy. Radiol Clin North Am. 2021;59(1):107–23.
7. Adrada BE, Miranda RN, Rauch GM, et al. Breast implant-associated anaplastic large cell lymphoma: radiologic findings and implications. Radiology. 2018;289(3):771–8.
8. Patel A, Bloom J, Nwariaku F, et al. Imaging findings after autologous fat transfer in breast reconstruction. Eur Radiol. 2023;33(2):1084–94.

Chapter 6
Axillary Findings on Chest CT in Patients with Breast Diseases

For the first assessment and screening of breast cancer, mammography is still the most used imaging modality. Depending on positioning and technique, the axillary region, especially the lower axilla, could be evaluated and it is possible to see some level I axillary lymph nodes on mediolateral oblique (MLO) images. Increased nodal density, loss of fatty hilum, cortical thickness, or asymmetric large nodes are all signs of suspicion. Mammography has a limited field of view which limits its sensitivity for a thorough axillary assessment. Because of this, mammography by itself is not enough to accurately assess axillary region [1, 2].

The main imaging technique for assessment of the axilla is ultrasound. Nodal morphology and vascularity can be assessed in real time and with great resolution. Normal lymph nodes are elliptical, with a thin cortex (usually less than 3 mm) and a preserved fatty hilum. Round shape, lack of hilum, eccentric cortical bulge, isolated or diffuse cortical thickening, and aberrant peripheral vascularity on Doppler imaging are all signs of suspicion. Ultrasound is essential to preoperative staging in patients with newly diagnosed breast cancer because it is particularly useful for directing core needle biopsy or fine-needle aspiration (FNA) of suspicious nodes. Ultrasound is operator dependent and has limitations when it comes to assessing deeper nodes in higher axillary levels, despite its advantages [3, 4].

Anatomically, the axilla is classified into three levels according to how it relates to the pectoralis minor muscle. This classification is crucial for both surgical and imaging evaluation.

- The level I nodes are situated inferior and laterally to the pectoralis minor muscle.
- The level II nodes are situated behind the pectoralis minor.
- The level III nodes are located medially and superior to the pectoralis minor.

This categorization has significant therapeutic and prognostic consequences for the stage of breast cancer. The majority of metastatic spread starts with level I nodes and works its way up. Deeper level II and III node involvement is better assessed by

A. Alikhassi, *Atlas of Breast Lesions on Chest Computed Tomography*,
https://doi.org/10.1007/978-3-032-22791-1_6

cross-sectional imaging modalities like CT and MRI, whereas ultrasound primarily analyzes level I and a portion of level II nodes [5, 6].

Chest CT is an important part of a thorough oncologic examination, but it is not often the first-line modality for axillary staging in early breast cancer. All three nodal levels, the supraclavicular areas, the internal mammary chains, and the mediastinum can be seen cross-sectionally with CT. Asymmetry relative to the contralateral side, uneven borders, central necrosis, lack of fatty hilum, and nodal enlargement (usually >1 cm short-axis diameter) are all signs of suspicious CT results. In oncologic imaging, CT provides a "one-stop-shop" benefit. CT can assess the initial breast mass to some extent, axillary nodal disease, lung metastases, pleural involvement, liver lesions, and osseous structures all in one examination. When a patient has incidental axillary lymphadenopathy, inflammatory breast cancer, or advanced disease, this thorough evaluation is especially helpful. CT is essential in some clinical situations because it can offer whole-body context, even though it is not as sensitive as ultrasound for subtle cortical changes in small lymph nodes [7, 8].

Figures 6.1, 6.2, 6.3, 6.4, 6.5, 6.6, 6.7, 6.8, and 6.9 demonstrate how chest CT scans are used to evaluate the axillary region in patients with breast diseases.

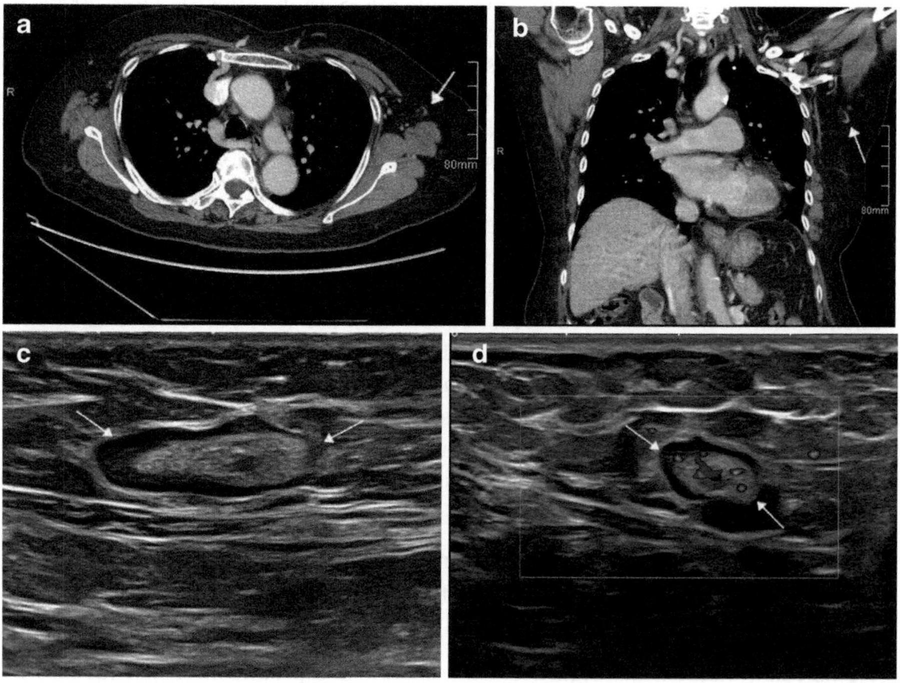

Fig. 6.1 Normal axilla. Chest CT with IV contrast axial (**a**) and coronal views (**b**), grayscale ultrasound (**c**), and color Doppler ultrasound (**d**). In a normal axilla on a chest CT scan, usually a few lymph nodes with preserved normal oval shape, a fatty hilum, and a thin cortex can be seen. In these images, a typical normal lymph node has been shown (solid arrow). On ultrasound of the same patient, a typical normal node with a thin cortex (<3 mm), an echogenic hilum, and an oval shape is seen. In the color Doppler interrogation, vascularity is only seen in the hilum, representing afferent and efferent vessels. There is no neovascularization of the cortex, which is characteristic of an infiltrated node

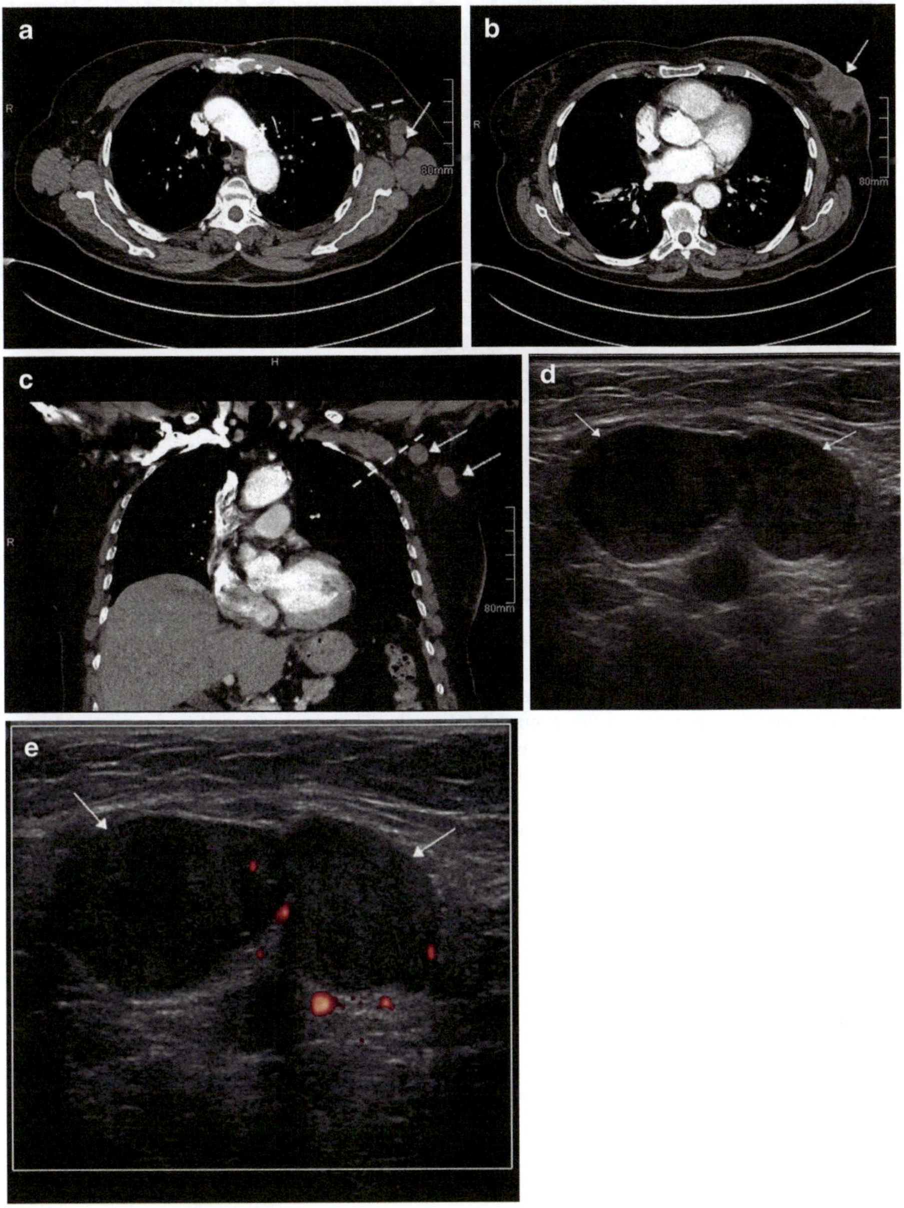

Fig. 6.2 Axillary level 1 lymph node metastasis. Chest CT with IV contrast axial (**a, b**) and coronal views (**c**), grayscale ultrasound (**d**) and color Doppler ultrasound (**e**) of a woman with known left breast invasive breast cancer, which had a staging chest CT scan. On the left axilla on the chest CT scan, two adjacent enlarged lymph nodes with a roundish shape, central low density, and no appreciable fatty hilum (solid arrow) are seen. The nodes are located lateral to the pectoralis minor muscle border (dashed line), which indicates level one nodes. The known cancer in the central breast involving nipple areolar complex and associated with central breast skin thickening is noted on image b (arrow). Ultrasound findings are consistent with the CT scan findings and show a bilobed, hypoechoic, and solid axillary mass with no appreciable fatty hilum, and with some peripheral vascularity suggestive of an infiltrated, conglomerated node

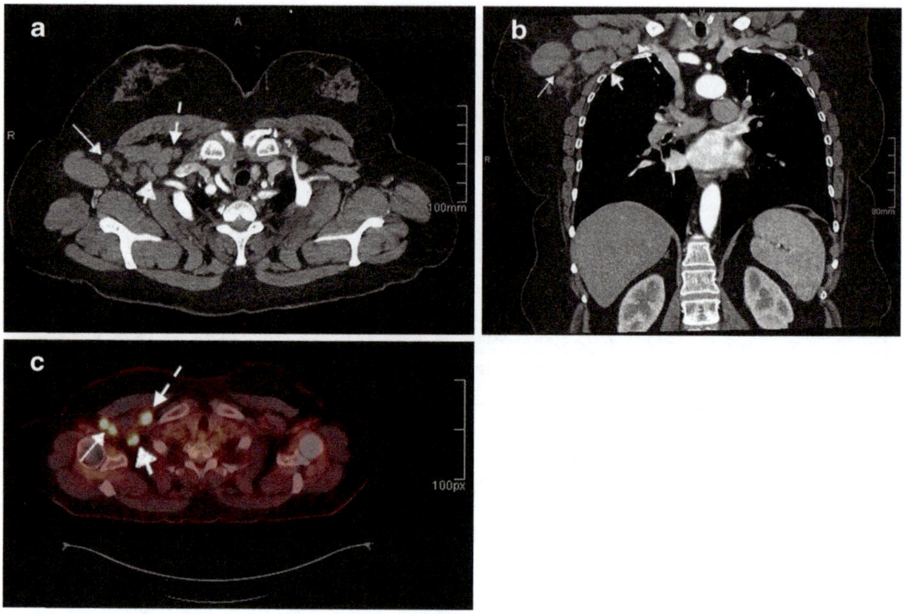

Fig. 6.3 Axillary level 2 and 3 lymph nodes metastasis. Chest CT with IV contrast axial (**a**) and coronal (**b**), FDG-PET CT scan (**c**) of a woman with known right breast advanced invasive breast cancer. On the right axilla, multiple enlarged, roundish lymph nodes with effaced fatty hilum are seen, asymmetric compared to the contralateral axilla. The abnormal nodes are scattered in all three axillary nodes as follows: lateral and inferior to the pectoralis minor muscle (level 1, solid arrow), posterior to the pectoralis minor muscle (level 2, thick short arrow) and superior medial to the pectoralis minor muscle (level 3, dashed arrow). The PET findings parallel with those of the chest CT scan and the nodes show avid uptake. One of the nodes in level 1 underwent ultrasound-guided core needle biopsy, which came back as malignant, consistent with known breast cancer metastasis

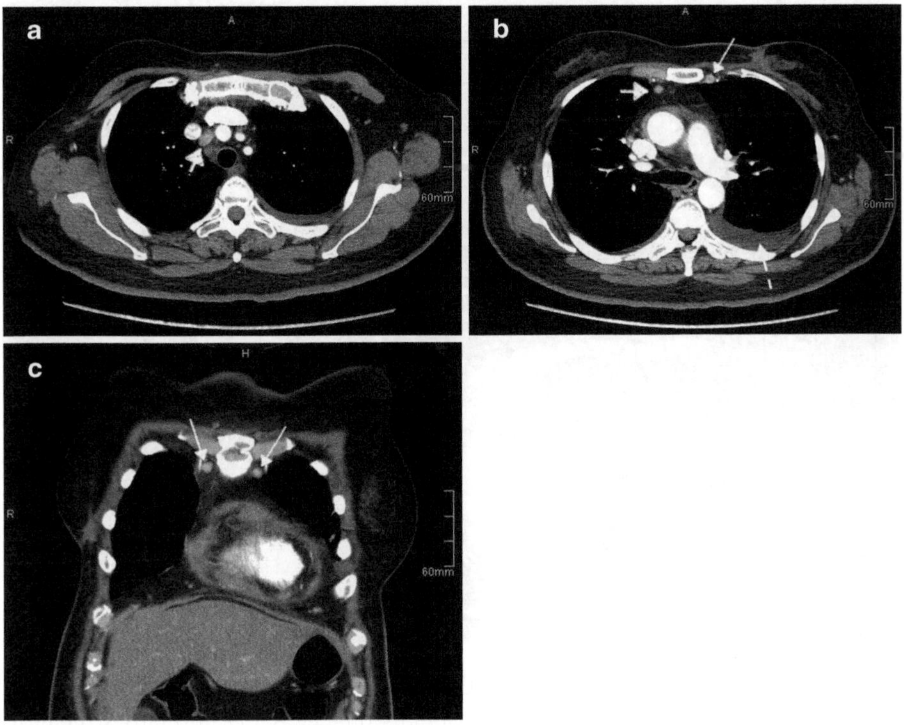

Fig. 6.4 Internal mammary lymph nodes metastasis. Chest CT with IV contrast axial (**a, b**) and coronal views (**c**) of a woman with a history of known metastatic right breast cancer. There are new slightly prominent, roundish lymph nodes in the mediastinum (short, thick arrow) and bilateral internal mammary chains (solid arrow). Additionally, there is a left side pleural effusion (dashed arrow) with positive cytology results for malignancy

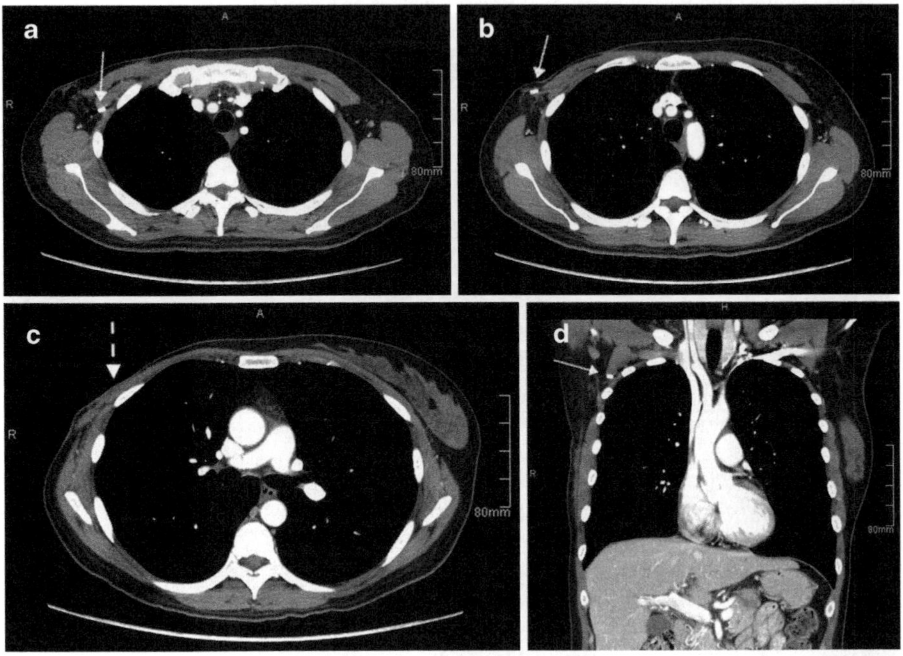

Fig. 6.5 Axillary dissection. Chest CT with IV contrast axial (**a–c**) and coronal views (**d**) of a woman with a history of right breast cancer who underwent a mastectomy and axillary dissection. In the right axilla, the CT scan reveals some stranding in the fatty tissue along with surgical clips, which indicate a previous axillary dissection (solid arrow). The signs of the mastectomy are more clearly visible in image **c** (dashed line)

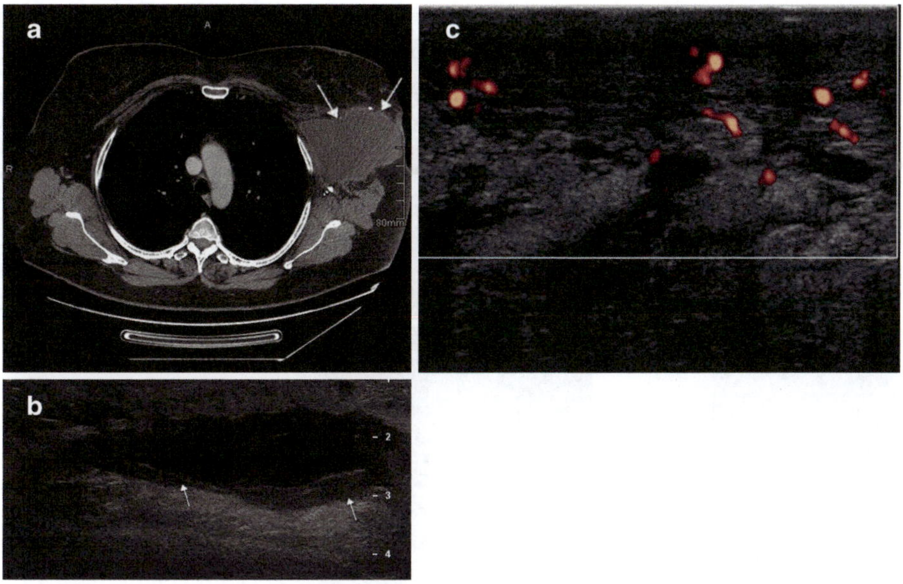

Fig. 6.6 Axillary complicated seroma. Chest CT with IV contrast axial view (**a**), grayscale ultrasound (**b**), and color Doppler ultrasound (c) woman with a recent history of left breast lumpectomy and limited axillary dissection presented with an axillary lump and overlying skin thickening. Chest CT scan revealed a large collection with fluid density in the left axilla, extending to the breast tail (arrows). Targeted ultrasound of the area showed a large fluid accumulation at the surgical site (arrows), accompanied by overlying skin thickening and increased vascularity on the color Doppler images, suggestive of inflammation. An ultrasound-guided aspiration was performed for both diagnostic and therapeutic purposes. The turbid yellow fluid obtained during the procedure was sent for smear and culture analysis. The results showed abundant inflammatory cells with no epithelial cells and a negative culture

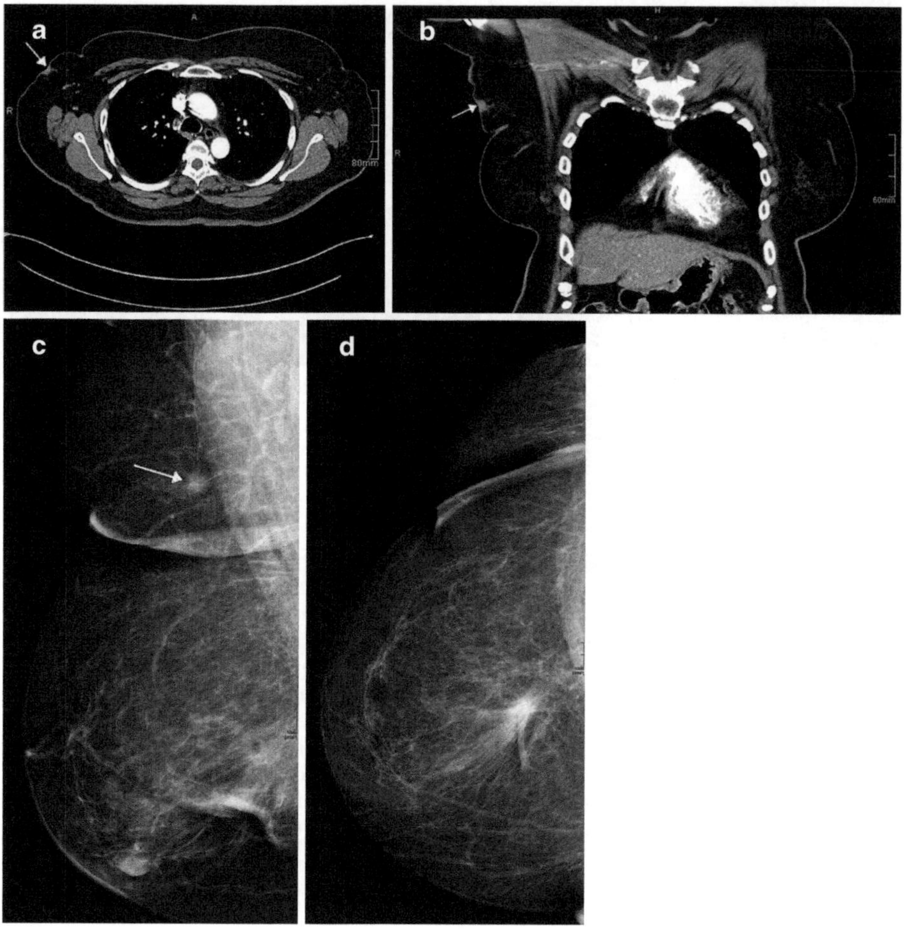

Fig. 6.7 Axillary tail recurrence. Chest CT with IV contrast axial (**a**), coronal views (**b**), mammography MLO view (**c**), CC view (**d**), gray scale ultrasound (**e**), and color Doppler ultrasound (**f**) woman with a history of right breast cancer and lumpectomy presented with an axillary tail lump. Chest CT scan revealed a right-sided superficial subdermal enhancing soft tissue mass in the axillary tail (arrows). Mammography demonstrates scar and signs of prior lumpectomy with a new subcentimeter soft tissue mass in the axillary tail, only included in MLO view, with no associated calcifications (arrow). Targeted ultrasound of the area showed a superficial heteroechoic vascular solid mass (arrows) with no posterior through transmission, which underwent a clinical punch biopsy with malignant results favoring recurrence. Differentiating benign skin lesions from dermal recurrences of breast cancer can sometimes be challenging. On ultrasonography, recurrence usually appears as an irregular, hypoechoic mass inside or just beneath the dermis with increased internal vascularity and indistinct borders. In mammogram, it is usually seen as a localized skin thickening or a new superficial mass. A benign dermal inclusion cyst, on the other hand, lacks internal vascularity in color Doppler evaluation unless it is inflamed, and it is usually oval, and circumscribed located within the dermis or subcutaneous layer with posterior acoustic enhancement on ultrasound. Clinical correlation is crucial, and biopsy is necessary when imaging findings are unclear

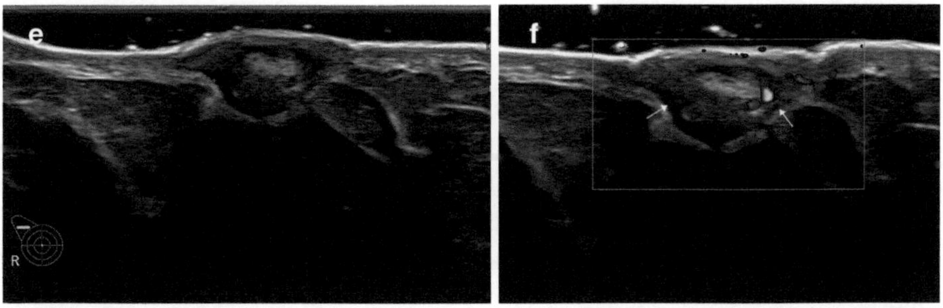

Fig. 6.7 (continued)

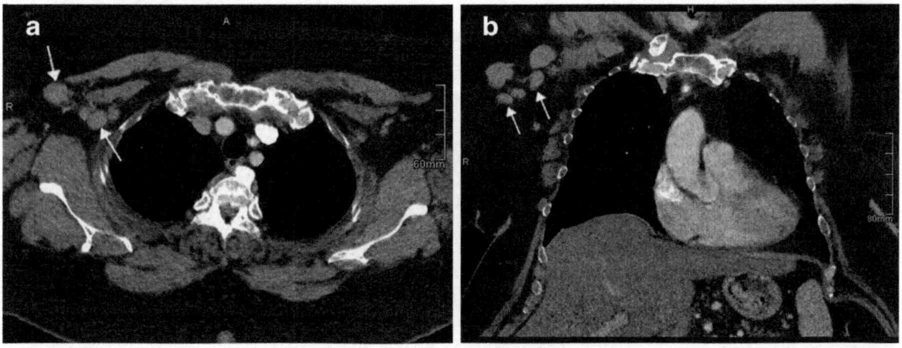

Fig. 6.8 Axilla in Systemic Lupus Erythematous. Chest CT with IV contrast axial (**a**), coronal views (**b**), mammography MLO spot views (**c, d**), gray scale ultrasound (**e**), and color Doppler ultrasound (**f**), woman with no history of present or prior breast cancer. Chest CT scan revealed asymmetric right-sided multiple enlarged axillary lymph nodes with no distinct fatty hilum (arrows). Spotted views of bilateral MLO view mammography are parallel with chest CT scan findings and show right-sided enlarged dense axillary nodes with no appreciable fatty hilum in some. In contrast, on the left, the lymph nodes are of low density and have a fatty hilum, typically benign (dashed arrow on image **d**). Targeted ultrasound of the right axilla demonstrates an enlarged lymph node (solid arrows) with significant cortical thickness and a small, squeezed echogenic fatty hilum (dashed arrow on image **e**) and scant vascularity in the hilum in the color Doppler evaluation (dashed arrow on image **f**). An ultrasound-guided core needle biopsy was performed, yielding reactive follicular hyperplasia, interfollicular expansion, and plasma cell infiltration, with no atypia or malignancy compatible with the patient's known history of SLE. Patient was advised of routine screening mammography, and axillary nodes' clinical and imaging follow-up

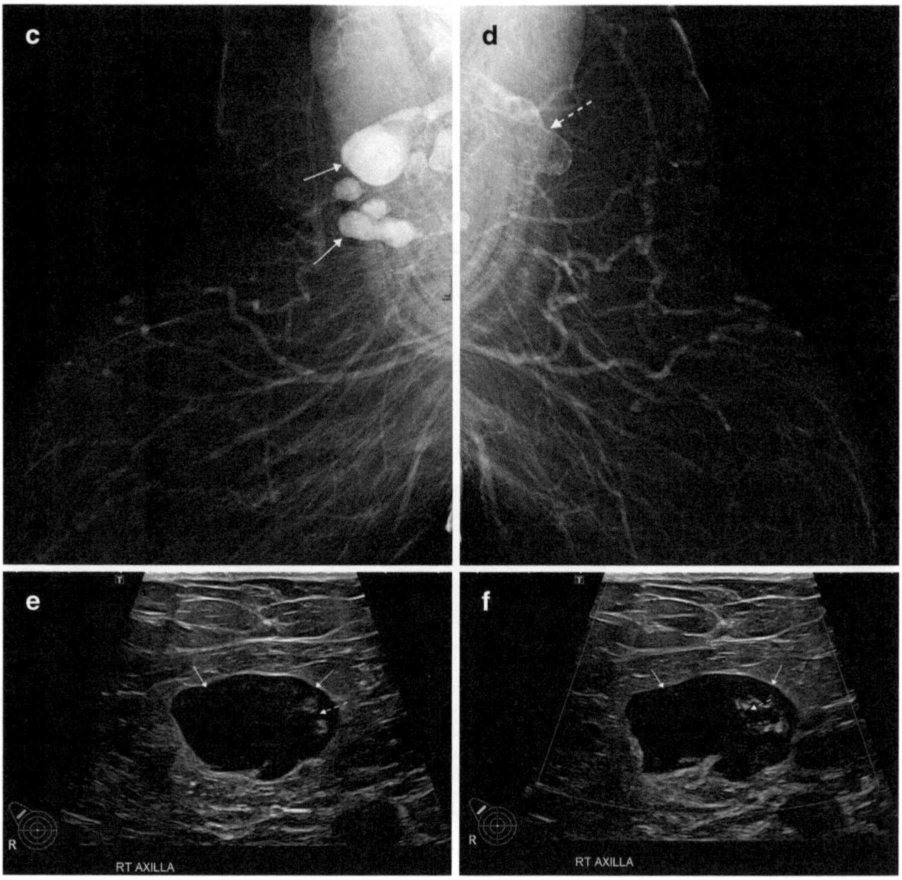

Fig. 6.8 (continued)

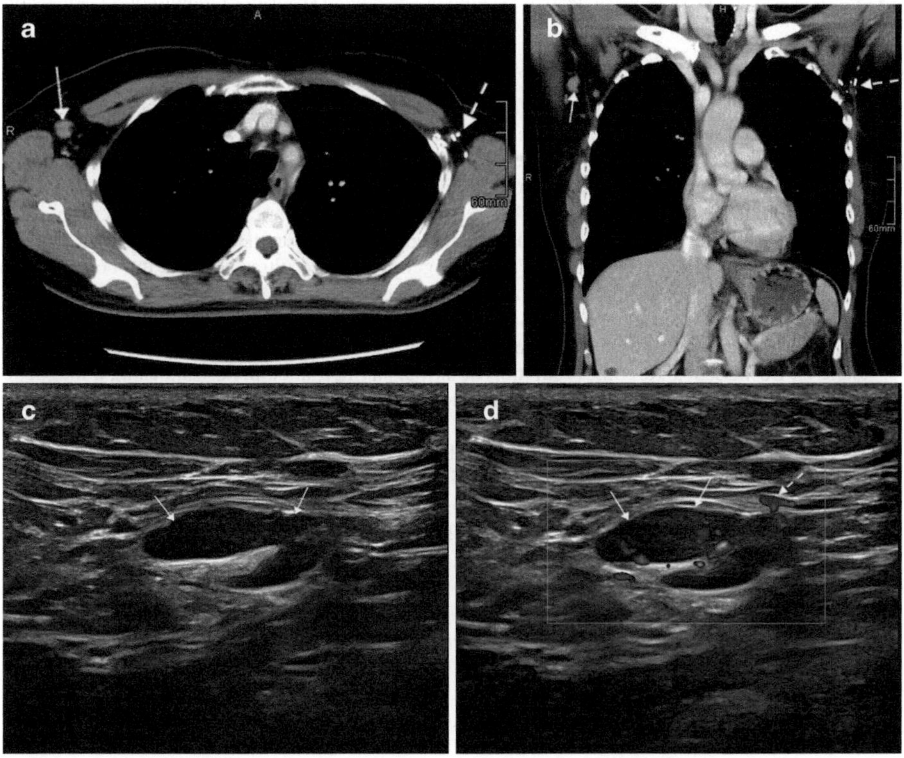

Fig. 6.9 Contralateral axillary metastasis. Chest CT with IV contrast axial (**a**), coronal views (**b**), gray scale ultrasound (**c**), and color Doppler ultrasound (**d**) of a woman with a history of previous left breast lumpectomy and left axillary dissection. Chest CT scan revealed a prominent right axillary lymph node with a small, squeezed, eccentric fatty hilum (solid arrow). In the left axilla, a few surgical clips are seen suggestive of signs of prior axillary dissection (dashed arrow). Targeted ultrasound of the right axilla demonstrates an enlarged lymph node (solid arrows) with cortical thickness above 3 mm and a squeezed echogenic fatty hilum. In the color Doppler evaluation, increased hilar vascularity and neovascularity outside the hilum close to the cortex (dashed arrow), suspicious for metastasis, are noted. The node underwent an ultrasound-guided core needle biopsy, which yielded malignancy. Differentials of metastasis from her known prior contralateral cancer and an unknown same side primary cancer were suggested, and a breast MRI was recommended which did not show a primary cancer in the right breast. Patient referred to the surgical and oncological team

References

1. Wang J, Di W, Shi K, Wang S, Jiang Y, Xu W, et al. Axilla view of mammography in preoperative axillary lymph node evaluation of breast cancer patients: a pilot study. Clin Breast Cancer. 2024;24(2):e51–60.
2. Teixeira SR, et al. Lymph node assessment in patients with early-stage breast cancer. RB Imagem. [Internet]. 2024; Available from: SciELO.
3. Moreth M, Herröder N, Hödl P, Bufe A, Bretschneider C, Möbus V, et al. Clinical axillary staging in breast cancer patients using ultrasound imaging. Breast Care (Basel). 2024;19(3):149–54.
4. Wang X, Nie L, Zhu Q, et al. Artificial intelligence assisted ultrasound for the non-invasive prediction of axillary lymph node metastasis in breast cancer. BMC Cancer. 2024;24:910.
5. Teixeira SRC. Axillary lymph nodes and breast imaging: limitations of mammography and advantages of cross-sectional evaluation. *RB Imagem* [Internet]. 2024; Available from: SciELO.
6. Jiang Z, Su Y, Zhang R, et al. Prediction of axillary lymph node metastasis using a magnetic resonance imaging radiomics model of invasive breast cancer primary tumor. Cancer Imaging. 2025;25:44.
7. Barszczyk M, Singh N, Bilbily A, et al. 3D CT radiomic analysis improves detection of axillary lymph node metastases compared to conventional features in locally advanced breast cancer. J Breast Imaging. 2024;6(4):397–406.
8. Systematic review on AI-based CT analysis of axillary lymph nodes. EJRAI. 2025;S3050-5771(25):00038–6.

Index

A. Alikhassi, *Atlas of Breast Lesions on Chest Computed Tomography*, https://doi.org/10.1007/978-3-032-22791-1

GPSR Compliance

The European Union's (EU) General Product Safety Regulation (GPSR) is a set of rules that requires consumer products to be safe and our obligations to ensure this.

If you have any concerns about our products, you can contact us on ProductSafety@springernature.com

In case Publisher is established outside the EU, the EU authorized representative is:

Springer Nature Customer Service Center GmbH
Europaplatz 3
69115 Heidelberg, Germany

Batch number: 10739801

Printed by Printforce, the Netherlands